Transdisciplinary Approaches to Healthcare Solutions during COVID-19

Edited by

Ravi Kant Avvari, Singam Jayanthu and Mohamed Sultan Mohamed Ali

Cambridge Scholars Publishing

Transdisciplinary Approaches to Healthcare Solutions during COVID-19

Edited by Ravi Kant Avvari, Singam Jayanthu and Mohamed Sultan Mohamed Ali

This book first published 2023

Cambridge Scholars Publishing

Lady Stephenson Library, Newcastle upon Tyne, NE6 2PA, UK

British Library Cataloguing in Publication Data
A catalogue record for this book is available from the British Library

ISBN (10): 1-5275-5094-X
ISBN (13): 978-1-5275-5094-0

TABLE OF CONTENTS

CHAPTER 1

OPHTHALMOLOGIC SOUNDINGS IN NEURO-FEEDBACK

JYOTIRMAYA SATPATHY[1], AHALYA HEJMADI[2], LIDIJA WEIS[3]

[1]Dept of Management and Leadership, Management University of Africa, Nairobi;
[2]Dept. of Behavioural Sciences & Psychology, University of Maryland Global Campus, Adelphi, (USA);
[3]Ljubljana School of Business, Ljubljana, Slovenia

ABSTRACT

Business 'decision - feedback sounding(s)' thinking has a biological basis. A paradigm for business leadership is emerging; a thinking business leader understands, develops, creates, engages and inspires. Business leaders end conventional thinking, understanding how to engage and influence the cerebral context and help activate openness to new ideas. In this, leaders' actions are transformed from results of a relationship orientation. This monograph aims to focus on the role of neuro-business in understanding business leadership strategy. The objective is to display the dynamics of neurobiological drivers in understanding behaviour. The aim is to understand empirical mosaics in 'neuro trajectory feedback sounding(s)' of 'business' decision circuit'. Relating to methodology, the monograph draws inspiration from business leadership and neuro-business works to evaluate the influence of the cerebral aspects in shaping communication, decision, negotiation, and emotion regulation that can directly be connected with business strategy. The study experiments to deduce causal knowledge. The methodology includes neuro-based opinions to imitate thinking of neurobiology in 'business' decision research. Based on a comprehensive literature review, models and prototypes, an eye-tracking experiment was conducted to measure eye positions (identifying fixations and saccades) and eye movement (geometry of stimulus). Results indicate a link between fixations, gaze and business decision-feedback sounding(s) thinking. The study provides key findings and explains how neuro-apparatuses explore 'business decision - feedback sounding(s)' thinking through biological basis in prototyping decision - feedback sounding(s) thinking. Results exhibit monikers to engage in 'business decision - feedback sounding(s)' thinking using eye-tracking techniques that business leadership delineate process information through activation of neuro-components. The monograph depicts the impact of biological processes as a significant element in business strategy. Activation of 'business decision - feedback sounding(s)' thinking processes helps interpret decision-making styles and how cerebral response to strategic 'business decision - feedback sounding(s)' thinking.

Keywords: *Neurobusiness; Business Leadership; Neuro Apparatuses; Decision - feedback sounding(s) Thinking and Strategic Leadership*

"If [philosophy of business] is worth doing at all, it must be done to gain new insights that will allow one to do better business" – Mittermaier, 1989.

1. INTRODUCTION

Leadership denotes the prospects of leading behaviour to achieve goals and objectives in an organisational setting. Leaders take an operative resolution to remove inconsistencies. Additionally, they are responsible for inspiring by signifying, backup and endeavouring to encourage positivity. Furthermore, it considers the organisation and its citizens' welfare and prosperity equally. Of late, there has been a lot of conversation around the future of the workroom, future-ready personnel, and the future of labour. As representatives of transformation, leaders have the serious character to perform in determining the future. In such a scenario, how can leaders grow future-ready workers? What could be the role of technology tomorrow? What inclinations would silhouette the ecosphere of labour? Organisational justice takes place from the perspective of consequentialist, functioning, cerebral and transactional interpretations in a multifaceted practice. At the same time, a move like this has been long overdue.

On the one hand, business is somewhat famous for its reluctance to discuss the path-dependent properties inherent in existing business stratification within regions, nations, and the world. Any change in this regard, and a more open consideration of the fact that today's discrepancies in wealth and opportunities in many cases derive from historical roots that relate to forced work and other atrocities of our past, would do us well to put things in an appropriate context. On the other hand, alternative theoretical perspectives are too often excluded based on mere prejudice, and any change in that regard is also to be applauded (Heterodox Business Newsletter, Issue. 297, May 30, 2022).

Business is civilisation, and unconventional business is current fruition. Neuro-entrepreneurial management sciences have linked disparate fields of management and psychology. Extension of microentrepreneurial management sciences counterparts advance of cognitive science. The interface between entrepreneurial business and brain sciences is not smooth, with misconceptions. Neuro-entrepreneurial discoveries posture a challenge to the usual management viewpoint. How can complexity in the philosophy of business leadership help advance the study of establishments, administration and revolution? What are the drivers of business leadership? How can the link between business leadership and pliability be inspected? How can organisations substitute pliability in a competitive setup? How can business leadership complexity philosophy aid in advancing performance? How can business leadership complexity philosophy procedures provision research? Why do some economies accomplish constant business growth while others miss the mark?

Curiosity in the radical economy, business expansion, business evolution and origination are correlated. An answer to this must be grounded on two masts: Radical Economy and Novelty. The world economy is moving inexorably towards a new phase, where large corporations will manage the purchase persuasion at will through new knowledge about the consumer's brain and big data tools. In this context, Neuro-business and Psychobusiness will become fundamental for the analysis of this new business world, where a deep scientific understanding of human emotions and feelings, both in consumption and in savings and investment, will nuance in a good way the ancient idea of "egotistical rationality", which from the hand of Adam Smith has been the cornerstone of the economy for more than two centuries. This extreme rationalist approach will no longer serve to understand the economy of the years to come. In this way, both business strategies and public policies will become neuro, incorporating everything that is known and will be known about the brain to better understand customers and voters. As a balance, business and political ethics will also become essential, given the excessive power of new neuro tools to influence people. The 21st Century will be the Century of the brain; say, many futurologists and business analysts will have to adapt to these changes (Laza and Marisela; 2021).

Growth is neither general nor undeviating leading to unwarranted social order. Are the working development replicas likely enough to create sustainability in evolution? How will the global business landscape assume its form in the 21st Century? What are the imposing undercurrents that would shape the destiny of business patterns? It is imperative to efficaciously endorse business progress, universal marketplace and provincial activities by abstracting a multifaceted structure finished by modest interrelating fragments. Complex systems are especially problematic to the rheostat. Computing these links can detect blockages to business advancements and shape the strategy towards a convergence pattern. Business 'decision - feedback sounding(s)' thinking has a biological basis. A paradigm for business leadership is emerging; a thinking business Leader understands, develops, creates, engages and inspires. Business leader appreciates, evolves, generates, engrosses and stimulates others through new insights and skills. Business Leaders end conventional thinking, understanding how to engage and influence the cerebral approach of others and help activate openness to new ideas. In this, Leader's actions are transformed from results orientation to relationship orientation. A precise understanding of the polycentric matrix is imperative to focus on the leadership aspect of decision-making progression. This invites a call for a changed and invigorated mindset, innovative dynamics in organisational order, and business leadership to comprehend and face competitive agents branded by other evidence and ecological subtleties.

2. LOCUS OF FOCUS

"It is true that humanity is faced with many problems. It always has been, but perhaps not always, with a such keen awareness of them as we have today. We might be more optimistic if we recognised that we do not have to solve all of these problems. Our essential task – a big enough one to be sure – is simply to keep open the options for the future or perhaps even to broaden them by creating new varieties and niches. Our grandchildren cannot ask more of us than we offer them the same chance for adventure, to pursue new and interesting designs." – Herbert Simon in The Sciences of the Artificial.

20th Century thinking stands outdated. Application of neuroscience in structural frameworks signifies a contour in field and laboratory experiments. Recapitulation of Cognito business as a human endeavour would merit clarification of substrates, instruments and flexible paraphernalia of emotional stimulus upon cognitive - feedback sounding(s) roles functioning in judgement-making progressions. Understanding human decision-making is currently a convergence of disciplines (psychology, neuroscience, and business) besides the synergy of methods (experimentation, cerebral imaging, and quantitative modelling). The human brain and eyes have always captivated humanity leading towards a cognitive - feedback sounding(s) revolution. How do cerebral dynamics evaluate knowledge and jeopardies? Under what neural mechanisms does it strike an equilibrium between constancy and framework sensitivity in decision, preferences and choice? What happens in the 'cerebral box' when (business) leaders style decisions or are in the process of making those? Is the study of Cognito business processes germane for business leaders? Does Cognito-business elucidate judgement-making, the potential to process multiple alternatives, and indicate an optimal course of action? Does Cognito-business study how business behaviour profile understanding of comprehensible cerebral undercurrents are causal to forecasting, regulating and decision making? These lead to the construction of a 'Cognito-business judgement-making inconsistency'. The goal is a conjecture of how cerebral apparatuses are tied to behaviour (Satpathy and Mund; 2022).

3. AIM AND OBJECTIVE

A paradigm for business leadership is emerging. The world is experiencing a thinking business leader who understands, develops, creates, engages and inspires. These leaders end conventional thinking, understanding how to engage and influence the cerebral of others and help activate openness to new ideas. In this, their actions are transformed from results orientation to relationship orientation. This monograph aims to focus on the role of neuro-business in understanding business leadership strategy. The primary aim is to archetype neuro-entrepreneurial neuro-feedback by using brain waves (EEG). This paper integrates neuro-entrepreneurial science and the psychology of management modelling tactics. The objective is to monitor neurobiological 'motorists' undercurrents in preference making. The effort is to elucidate how neural investigations appreciate 'mental sounding' in entrepreneurial decision-making. The pivotal point is to comprehend causal processes of how Entrepreneurs craft decisions, appreciate apparatuses of decision making and integrate interdisciplinary scholarship in the direction of a contributive neuro-entrepreneurial decision. The objective is to monitor the dynamics of neurobiological drivers in understanding business leadership behaviour via empirical mosaics in 'neuro trajectory feedback sounding(s)' of 'business' decision circuit'. As regards methodology, experimentation was run to measure eye positions (Identifying fixations and saccades) and eye movement (geometry of stimulus). Results indicate the link between fixations, gaze and business decision - feedback-sounding (s) thinking.

4. MOTIVATION

The foundation of stimuli has been neuro-entrepreneurial decision explorations (merger of philosophies from cognitive science and management). Neuro-entrepreneurial decision-making has arisen as an interdisciplinary determination to bridge this gap. It mixes ideas from organisational psychology, neuro-entrepreneurial science and neuro-entrepreneurial - management to stipulate precise representations of decision-making.

5. PROBLEM STATEMENT

Notwithstanding considerable developments, enquiry of how we make decisions stays to posture significant trials for methodical explorations. Erecting a decision infers that there is an alternate choice to be factored in. And in such a circumstance, we want not only to detect as many of these substitutions as conceivable but select the one that (1) has a peak prospect of efficiency and (2) best fits with the goal line, needs, routine, and ethics.

6. LITERATURE SCAN

The origin of Cognito business can be traced to 'Wealth of Nations' in 1776, which explains influenced behaviour, appreciating judgement behaviour and accumulation of judgements. One School of Thought was on regularities in behaviour that could (Ceteris Paribus) provide a psychological basis to manage business preferences. The Second School of Thought advocates sequences of theorems that protract revealed - preference philosophy to business leadership judgements. This is a period in which heterogeneous researchers have begun to develop models of mental processes and correlate intermediate variables. As a sign of globalisation, the world is swiftly becoming an integration of intercontinental frugality, trade, philosophy, policies and information. Thoughtful digital transformation, vicissitudes, and procedures, besides growth, skills and knowledge transfer, succeed as the potential frame for knowledge development, business consistency, affordability and development. For business leaders, promoting convergence in a field characterised by a high degree of complexity is morally significant. The question is, under what conditions would such functions exist (Satpathy and Mund; 2022)?

Balconi (2020) explained that neuro-management was born from a need to comprehend mental processes subserving motives, attitudes, and behaviours of professionals in organisations to predict, modify, and/or enhance. Quite a few argue that lack of familiarity with neuroscientific methods (Nofal; 2018), uncertainty about expectations (Murray and Antonakis; 2019), resistance compared to looking in the Black Box (Becker; 2011), and presence of ethical issues have made professionals of organisations rather cautious (Butler; 2016). Boone and Piccinini (2016) outlined that the cognitive feedback-sounding (s) neuroscience revolution consists of rejecting scientific practices stemming from the traditional two-level view of cognitive feedback-sounding (s) science and replacing them with a fully integrated science of cognition. Konovalov and Krajbich (2019) asked whether neuro-business kept its promises: "Unfortunately, finding analogous ties between brain regions and psychological constructs such as 'value' has proven more challenging." Grayot (2020) critically reviewed dual-process philosophy for human reasoning and decision-making in all neuro-thing literature. The focus is on deciphering such transactions and requires understanding Cognito processes that implement value-dependent judgment-making.

7. ULTIMATE TECTONICS

Human resources relies on sensitivities that facilitate information. The tactic involves building models to present the relationship between reason and Cognito absurdity. The freedom provided by the tactic primes to a model of a mental process (cognitive - feedback sounding(s) process) that leads to the selection of a path of action among alternatives. These replicate compensatory crossing points of business judgement, cerebral structure, approach, characters and outline. Consequently, business judgement is a reasoning or emotional development which can be rational or irrational. This leads to 'Cognito-business judgement making inconsistency'. These accede to how the cerebral encrypts, processes data, and stores representation to craft stimuli. These embrace consciousness and perception of data, interface linking data, protoplasmic arrangement (configuration) of memory and dispensation of data. In such a spectrum, neuro-business leadership plays the role of understanding the cerebral reason for behaviours. Key snags include how the cerebral characterises the value of diverse inclinations and capitulates the best possible business judgement-making. Which are the limits for test potential in experimentation? Could we experiment with business judgement-making flawlessly, mimicking valid contexts? Is top-down control involved? Do we have liberated will, and to what extent do we have room for inclination, if any? The fundamental limitation is that it can spot different cerebral regions in definite situations. All these intensify cognitive-feedback sounding(s) complexity.

In history, previous civilisations witnessed erudite business notions and inscribed leaders of the finest business practices and standards in the 1st millennium BCE. The first theoretical exposition was propounded by Tunisian philosopher Ibn Khaldun, writing in the 14th Century, who was among the first theorists to examine who dwelt on the separation of labour, revenue object and transnational trade. Adam Smith applied the philosophies of the French Enlightenment to advance on how frugality should work, followed by Karl Marx and Thomas Malthus expanded on his work. Statistics and mathematics were interjected by Walras and Marshall to prompt economies of scale. Keynes advanced theories to bring dynamism to monetary policy. Amartya Sen's reasons for factorisation of integrity in social wellbeing calculations of business competence. Currently, Industry 5.0 promises prodigious swings with the help of data science and IoT technologies. With a focus on the problem-solving and inventiveness, automation will team up with humans at diverse levels. Industry 5.0 envisions new business information and considerations that will transmute present trends. In such an arrangement, there is an unavoidable need to grow leadership aids, including problem resolution, directional, communication, tactical planning, solidarity, conflict steadfastness and time administration. This is to be complemented and supplemented with the introduction of professional issues from different establishments, bargain explanations using biofeedback sounding(s) and mentoring the next cohort of practitioners and investigators to support best practices that add value to the comprehensive profession.

Real-life decision-making encompasses the calculation of the induced value of various actions by reasoning and expressive processes. Leaders have a vision-backed mission. Ancient models of leadership have changed. There has been a paradigm shift. New models have gone over the properties of augmented VUCA. New-fangled critical neuro-business leadership competencies are setting in. The concentration of a leader is on delivering transformational consequences. Leaders need to focus principally on strengths and on cultivating weaknesses. Leaders need to be resolve-obsessed ('moonshots' purpose). However, situations often require judgements between many complex and conflicting alternatives, with a high degree of uncertainty and ambiguity. The goal is to make better and 'rational' business judgement making. Theories and prescriptions require a cognitive - feedback sounding(s) understanding of business leadership business behavioural judgement system. The question of appropriate prescriptions is directed towards the conceptualisation of business leadership and business behaviour equipped with implications for understanding strategy. Some business leadership business behaviour fails to achieve the goals of the firm. One way of looking at it is a pre-existing framework of conceptualisation and analysis can be resolved with the initial judgement process. It also has to be recognised that once strategic judgements have been made, and a suitable judgement framework is established, then the business leadership work involved in such decisions becomes increasingly routine. The objective will be to reach an acceptable balance so that judgement is made promptly and coordinated. The operational measure of balance/imbalance between neural systems is the extent of temporal discounting apparent in a business leader's Cognito judgement behaviour. This ensures that conflict between goals is minimised. The explanation has often concentrated on functional and dysfunctional Cognito judgement business leadership business behaviour (Satpathy and Mund; 2022).

8. EXPERIMENTATION: RESULTS AND DISCUSSION

Human choices define human beings. How to introduce a 'human-centric choice'? In fact, what is a human-centric choice? Is it a beginning or end to a specific contemplation? Do they have a biological basis? Do these have bio - computational philosophical connotations? Are they regulated by some genetic 'drivers' like human sense organs? Such an archetype is concerned with perception underpinning a driver's choice. If yes, then who serves as a 'driver'? Leadership replicas are concomitant with technical novelty. Voyaging through 'bust-amination' ('businesses and 'contamination'), the leadership community is transversely at cater - cornered with neuroscience and entrepreneurship, transmitting a perceptive organised linkage ('Chess Board Matrix'). Key regeneration originates with rational information as 'control'. The final question is: are these networked neurologically ('neural roulette')? This amounts to 'rationality'. Do these represent a sweeping renaissance of primary concerns in understanding the biology of choice apparatus?

Eye movements are connected to optical deliberation as leading tools for electing stimulating dividends of chromatic projections for augmented perceptual and rational processing. Examination of leadership decision-making has protracted from the leadership decision behaviourist approach to the cerebral approach, which focuses on decision processes. The problem statement is that, in eye simulations, the choice is represented by spots of neural activity linked to stimulating prospects for rational processing that help acquisition, possessing and sketching leadership choice formation replicating computational choice formation.

9. METHODOLOGY AND DESIGN PARAMETERS

Eye-tracking choice research, through neuro-ocular approaches is distinguished by the occurrence of collaborating solicitations. Eye movements are an integral part of interactions with the ocular world. This is for inspecting the contents of a neuro-ocular scene or navigating through the environment. This brings eyes quickly and accurately to important positions. Eye movements accomplish this without external stimulation or spontaneous and self-generated activity. This manifests itself as oscillations in different frequency bands. Research explores the effect of neuronal oscillation perceptual processes (amplification or filtering) that cannot be observed directly. Instead, they can be identified by modelling empirical 'inferential' data with models. These explain the relationship between functional methodologies, experimental conditions and emotional 'inferential' data. With different disciplines approaching through characteristically different techniques and substantial advances, the question of how leaders design business choices has engaged scholars for decades (Satpathy, 2015).

10. RESEARCH DESIGN

The objective was to learn about relevant eye tracking, design research questions, tasks and possible metrics, test stimulus, create tests, analyse tracking 'inferential' data and generate result deliverables. Subjects were briefed about the experiments and were provided with 'material' on which they were to be tested as regards their comprehension of the provided information. The principal objective of the experiment was to contribute to the neuro-ocular domain with accepted optimal techniques. The aim was to have a 'cognitive - feedback sounding(s) - link' with 'heat maps' to connect neuro-ocular information schema. Heat maps were adopted to answer the questions about what fascinates participants' responsiveness (**Fig. 2**). How does one look at a spot when undertaking a task? How do subjects allocate attention over an inducement? These helped connect important aspects of neuro–ocular information graphic behaviour. Gaze plots were observed as crucial contributions in the neuro-ocular domain with accepted optimal techniques that set potential benchmarks for business choice-making. All these experimental designs aimed to understand and inquire if a relationship exists between how subjects assimilated information and understanding of 'material' information.

To confirm that the eye-tracking experiment was correctly inferred and simulated, the experiment atmosphere, the geometry of light settings, the geometry of stimulus, font of 'material', system configuration, population traits, regulation corroboration method, timing, 'inferential' data route, AOIs and segregation criteria were defined. After the Area of Interest was restricted, 'inferential' data was transferred to eye-tracking software (Tobii) for each AOI. Eye movements were conducted to include fixations (when the eye stops and focuses) and saccades (when the eye moves between fixation points). Eye movements were undertaken to have fixations (when the eye stops and focuses) and saccades (when the eye moves between fixation points).

Design emphasis was to;

- Articulate queries and primary style observations,
- Articulate supposition and make likelihoods,
- Choose developmental methods and research strategy,
- Outline each measure,
- Select suitable recorded 'shots' technique,
- Practice recorded 'shots' technique,
- Collect facts and develop 'Heat Maps', and
- Analyse information to draw inferences.

Experiments were piloted at the Fang Yang Laboratory, Graduate Institute of Science Education, New Taiwan Normal University, Taipei, Taiwan, to resemble a typical choice-oriented setting. Subjects were tested on their comprehension of VUCA information. Tobii Eye Sensor was used for neuro-ocular purposes. The literature manual from Tobii Company illustrates that depending on system design, Tobii uses different NIR sensors and illuminators. Tobii Eye Sensors offer specific sensors and illuminators for each neuro-ocular design. Tobii uses imperceptible near-infrared light and tall classification cameras to assign light to the leadership eye. Then, it registers the path they are revealed. After that, sophisticated algorithms calibrate eyes and regulate foci on which where they are convexed. Tobii combines custom-designed and standard components typically used in higher-volume designs.

- **F1** – Displays live view to help place subject.
- **F2** – Perform a simple one-point standardisation update.
- **F3** – Launch full standardisation.

- **F4** – Pointers become imperceptible.
- **F5** – Introduction of locations edge.
- **F6** – Hides hotspot at top.
- **F7** – Recesses eye-tracking.
- **F8** – Clasp left click lock.
- **F9** – Quick access exit.

11. RESEARCH STRATEGY

As this research (neuro-ocular) is a maiden attempt within the spectrum of neuro management, observed as crucial contributions in its neuro-ocular domain with accepted optimal techniques that set potential benchmarks for business choice-making, it is prudent to place an extract from Tobii manual (**Fig. 1**).

Thirty (30) healthy volunteer respondents were accorded space for undertaking the tests. New Taiwan Normal University, Taipei approved all experimental procedures. At the start of each experiment session, a 'material' was provided to the subject to be read aloud and then a silent reading. After that, the Lab entrepreneur in the station regulated the eye tracker for each participant to map 'points' on the monitor. After calibration, participants' references were captured, reflecting the perception of cognitive – feedback sounding(s) load. 'Inferential' data were collected for each contributing subject independently. The stimuli, procedures, and analyses used in experiments were designed and deliberated at Fang Ying convened Eye-tracking Lab, New Taiwan Normal University, Taipei. Some operational details were obtained directly from Prof Fang Ying convened. Subjects differentiated upward from downward motion, and random dot impetuses were located to the left and/or right of fixation. Visual stimuli were created and considered. This was done using a Pentium – class computer operating within a Windows XP environment. Visual stimuli were displayed using a linearised 42″ CRT monitor. It had an animated rate of 60 Hz. The screen was viewed by subjects from a distance of 65cm. A chin rest was used. This was to steadily observe the situation. All experiments were performed in a dimly-illuminated testing booth. Test results are presented in subsequent section(s) subtitled 'Results' below.

> 'Eye-tracking analysis is based on the important assumption that there is a relationship between fixations, gaze and thinking. The spatial and Temporal sampling ability of the eye limits the manner to extract ocular information from events. However, because ocular acuity decreases when we move away from the centre of the ocular field, we possess a repertoire of eye movements that allow eyes at target locations of interest. Fixations are common features of looking that eye-tracking researchers analyse to make inferences about cognitive - feedback sounding(s) processes or states they are interested in probing. Fixations are those times when eyes essentially stop scanning the scene, holding central fovea vision in place so that the ocular system can take in detailed information about what is being looked at. But how do we get fixations? Fixations are constructions and outputs of a mathematical algorithm that translates the sequence of raw gaze points into an associated sequence of fixations.

Fig. 1: An extract from the Tobii manual

12. OBSERVATIONS AND DISCUSSIONS

'Inferential' data from each subject were analysed independently. Error rates were quite low even with the MSS (memory set size) of 100 objects. Observations were correct 85% of the time. There was a main effect of both presence of the target item and MSS on response accuracy: target presence, $F\ (1, 12) = 31.18$, $p < 0.001$, generalised eta squared (g-η2), a measure of effect size) = 0.25; MSS, $F\ (1.44, 18.85) = 88.80$, $p < 0.001$, g-η2 = 0.51, and the two factors interacted significantly, $F\ (1.47, 19.30) = 23.77$, $p < 0.001$, g-η2 = 0.04. Real-time 'inferential' data on correct references follow the same pattern of large main effects for both factors: target presence, $F\ (1, 12) = 28.71$, $p < 0.001$, g- η2 = 0.24; MSS, $F\ (1.37, 17.88) = 83.81$, $p < 0.001$, g-η2 = 0.51, and substantial interaction between the two, $F\ (2.46, 31.94) = 24.26$, $p < 0.001$, g-η2 = 0.04. The slope was significantly influenced by target presence, $F\ (1, 12) = 37.25$, $p < 0.001$, g-η2 = 0.27. In addition, there was a significant effect of MSS on the search slope, $F\ (1.33, 17.47) = 45.43$, $p < 0.001$, g-η2 = 0.45. In sum, behavioural results are in substantial agreement with previous work. There was a significant effect of target presence (all F values > 7, $p < 0.04$) on all measures except dwell time on fixated distractors, $F\ (1, 12) = 2.00$, $p = 0.17$, g-η2 = 0.01. In all cases, two factors interacted such that the effect of target presence became larger as MSS increased (all Fs > 5, all ps< 0.004). The percentage of distractors fixated on absent references increases significantly from an average of 22% per O per reference to 72% as MSS increases from one to 100 items, $F (1.74, 22.87) = 56.9$, $p < 0.001$, $g\text{-}\eta 2 = 0.55$. Dwell time on each distractor rose from 52 to 290 ms, $F (1.24, 16.23) = 27.97$, $p < 0.001$, $g\text{-}\eta 2 = 0.36$. This result replicates if we restrict the analysis to only fixated distractors, $F (1.27, 16.57) = 13.55$, $p < 0.004$, $g\text{-}\eta 2 = 0.23$. Total fixations per item on absent references rose from 0.26 with one item in memory to 1.27 with 100 items in memory, $F (1.26, 16.32) = 29.23$, $p < 0.001$, $g\text{-}\eta 2 = .36$. Fixations could be interpreted in different ways depending on context and objective of the study. During the processing of the neuro-ocular scene, individuals moved their eyes to relevant features in that scene. The peripheral area primarily detected some features. Based on this, it can be inferred that 'leadership choice making is unswerving inter-oriented to instantaneous accessibility and effortlessness of analysis of pertinent 'material' evidence'. Neurophysiological experiments reveal that neurons in the prefrontal cortex display saccade–oriented activity. Saccade–oriented activity in the prefrontal cortex shows steering discernment and setting dependence. Inherent characteristics are parallel between pre/post-saccadic activities. The above results indicate the prefrontal cortex and eyes might contribute to saccadic eye movements. This does play a role in cognitive – feedback sounding(s) functions or monitoring leadership behaviour.

The results above lend credence to the aim of experiments undertaken, in that eye-tracking methodology does help in investigating and corroborating dynamics of leadership choice-making. Results exhibit an essential link between 'subjective', 'physiological' and 'fixations' from a real-world point of view. When leaders make choices, there's a heavy disparity in comportment. 'Vacillating' leaders employ additional evidence when attempting an option compared to 'definite' leaders. First, there were differences in the manner leaders scanned available information. While 'definite' leaders spot on to a choice based on a particular trait, 'vacillating' leaders take in all of the 'material'. 'Definite' leaders perhaps opine that all options have 'good' and 'bad' characteristics. But they prefer a feature that is presumably important. 'Vacillating' leaders observed and opined that all 'materials had some quota of 'good' and 'bad' points. Secondly, 'vacillating' individuals distributed available time over a greater number of attributes during their course of experimental observation. The 'definite' participants 'focused' on fewer attributes to make their choice. Interestingly, 'vacillating' leaders spent more time overall looking at nothing. The subjects looked at 'blank cells' in the 'grid' while (apparently) attempting to make a choice. This series of experiments theorises that undertaking leaders to 'cogitate' or 'reframe' selections before arriving at a choice.

Prefrontal neurons display saccade–oriented action. Appreciating how the leadership brain works is significant in footings of meaningful impact on cognitive – feedback sounding(s) functions. Pre-saccadic activity encrypts guidelines of eye movements. The brain filters out unwanted information when leaders shift vision from one target to another focal target. The complexity of (leadership) 'intended' choice problems increases with the options and features of each available option. Neuro-intended choice, from eye-tracking processes (images and responses) to complex results, makes assumptions about how (leaders) make intended choices and defines the link between (leadership) choices and (leadership) preferences. This postulates that leaders fully understand the 'intended' choice problem and adopt optimising behaviour to create 'intended' choices. Neuro–ocular action towards leadership-oriented behaviour, capable of explaining leadership choice making, on cognitive – feedback sounding(s) models of choice, recommends the following;

- Escape from clichés and arrangements,
- Challenge conventions,
- Generate options and alternatives,
- Strategies new designs and observe what happens, and
- Find new access opinions from which to change forward.

13. INFERENCE

Neuro–ocular analysis is based on the assumption that there is a relationship between fixations, gaze and what leaders consider in matters of choice. Insistently, the prefrontal cortex of the leadership brain is responsible for visual stability. Eye-tracking techniques reveal the ability to aid in leadership choice dynamics. Settings, lengths and records in prechosen 'areas of interest' with transitions indicate 'degree of attention allocation' to prechosen areas. These exhibit how choice-making can be explored with eye-tracking techniques. However, it reflects methodological concerns when interpreting 'inferential' data. Research needs renewed thinking and undertaking things to address them. Primarily, sometimes fixations do not necessarily translate into conscious cognitive – feedback sounding(s) process. For example, during a search task, one can easily fixate briefly on a search object and miss its presence, especially if an object has an unexpected shape or size. These happen in the form of expectations of what objects should look like, modulating ocular attention and further interference with object detection. As an inference, the above study attempts to explore phenomena through neuro–ocular action, management-oriented choice and reasoning processes on cognitive feedback sounding(s) models of choice. This provides a framework for understanding and conducting research at the intersection of brain–and eye–based models capable of predicting management–oriented behaviour capable of explaining leadership choice-making.

Eye-tracking measures provide non-invasive indices of brain dynamics. Gaze examination divulges attentional and cognitive – feedback sounding(s) approaches. Ocular measures deliver perceptions concerning cognitive

- feedback sounding(s) expanses. As a concluding note to this Chapter, this thesis advocates auxiliary inquiries to scan physiognomies of saccade–related dynamics in the prefrontal cortex and the conceivable influences on eye movement mechanism and related – prefrontal functions. Eye-tracking offers a novel peep into choice management.

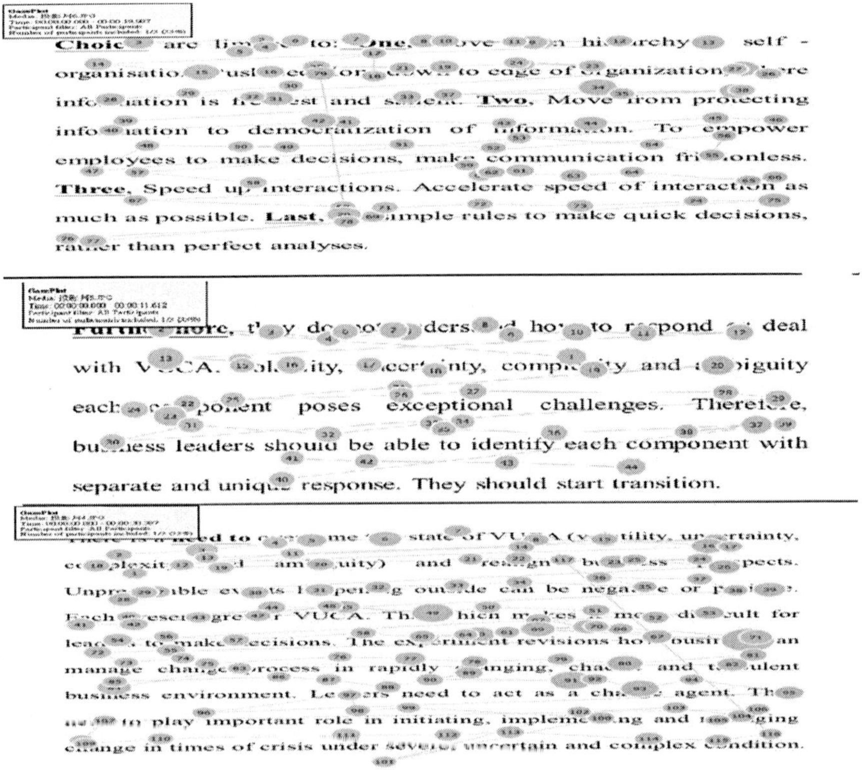

Fig. 2: Heat maps from one of the analysis

14. CONCLUSION

Making cogent psychosomatic decisions in a state of Chaos and Resilience is a management action. Cerebral Science (Cerebral Management) has made advances, bringing unprecedented insights into the human brain and decision-making. Inquiry is witnessing multilevel research in organisational studies integrating delineated research domains and offering a novel lens for understanding business practice. Human organisations are at a crossroads between cerebral and business laying a conduit that seems an abnormal approximation with infinite 'Scrolling', Chaos, Complexity and 'Interpolations'. The impression that decisions are taken through rational or logical thought processes has been exposed to questioning by experiments that analyse estimation during decision-making. Reference is drawn to bio-processes that impact decisions, activate to differentiate based on multiple signals of origin, and conditions that support or negate findings that aid understanding how neuro-configurations influence decision-making. Documentation of molecular and genetic markers precisely forecast rational physiognomies for understanding neural mechanisms of 'Chaos' and 'Resilience' in leadership decision-making.

Are 'business actors' being threatened by 'decision alarm'? 'Business actors' assume that decisions are rational, optimal and based on the best accessible data. They postulate that they totally appreciate decision-feedback-sounding (s) behaviours. Such propositions are now scanned under the lens of cellular and chromosomal prisms. Issues like how decision-feedback sounding(s) processes transgress in brain pathways, how the brain considers data sources and what intrinsic processes embody conflicting 'Chaos' and' Resilience' values have been explored to design 'rational' decisions. The objective has been to monitor the philosophy of neurobiological drivers in behavioural models towards understanding neurobiological drivers that underlie behaviour and decision-making using fundamental tools from business, psychology, neuroscience, mathematics and statistics. The significant finding is that business actor attempts to decide and evaluate prospective decision in Chaos and Resilience conditions using blood glucose medium and eye-tracking.

Leaders (Actors) contract high uncertainty, ambiguity, time pressure and emotional stress. Neural mechanisms of behavioural strategy-based sustainable decision-making require the integration of evidence over time until a response threshold is reached. Cognito - management investigates behavioural strategy-based sustainable decision-making using 'Cognito - Tactical Monikers' (CTM) to investigate how the brain behaves in the circuit of higher cognitive - feedback sounding(s) functions. This has transitioned from mapping confined effects, to evolving extrapolative models that assimilate data scattered across brain structures. In a progressively complex management milieu, leaders struggle between tactical arrangements and precise methods to gauge the degree of accomplishment of predetermined goals. Behavioural strategy-based sustainable decision-oriented planning assists as a 'catalyst' in cognitive - feedback sounding(s) behaviours. There is a need to understand behavioural-biological 'drivers' for investigating underlying behavioural - mechanisms of sustainable decision processes. The scope is to know how leadership trait mapping divulges behavioural insight. The factual lateral lies in analysing available verifiable, reliable and significant information, filtering and sieving of available data and accessing expressive information. This is supplemented by actions of behavioural compartments to further process interactive-oriented actions. In neural computational simulations, the decision is represented by a node of neural motion encompassing mechanisms of spiralling of activity and initiation for the neural motion to scan positioning of eye movements as a fundamental rationale of leadership decision.

REFERENCES

1. Kowler, E. (1989). Cerebral expectations, not habits, control anticipatory smooth oculomotor pursuit. Journal of Vision Research, 29, 1049-1057, USA.
2. Kowler, E. (1990). (Ed.) Eye Movements and their Role in Visual and Cerebral Process. Volume 4 in Reviews of Journal of Oculomotor Research, Elsevier Science Publishers, Amsterdam.
3. Kowler, E. (1990). The role of visual and cerebral processes in the control of eye movement. In Eye Movements and Their Role in Journal of Visual and Cerebral Processes. (Edited by Kowler, E.) Elsevier, Amsterdam.
4. Kowler, E. (1991). The stability of gaze and its implications for vision. In Journal of Eye Movements (Volume 9 of Vision and Visual Dysfunction) (Edited by Carpenter, R.H.S.). Macmillan Press, London.
   http://www.rci.rutgers.edu/~kowler/fixation1991.pdf
5. Kowler, E. (1995) Cogito ergo move: Cerebral eye movement control. In Exploratory Vision: The active eye. (Edited by Landy, M., Maloney, L. And Pavel, M.) Springer-Verlag, USA.
6. Kowler, E. (1995) Eye movement. In: Invitation to Cerebral Science, Vol. 2. (Edited by Kosslyn, S.). MIT Press, USA.
7. Kowler, E. And Blaser, E. (1995). The accuracy and precision of saccades to small and large targets. Vision Research, 35, 1741-1754, USA.
8. Kowler, E. And Sperling, G. (1980). Transient stimulation does not aid visual search: Implications for the role of saccades. Journal of Perception and Psychophysics, 27, 1-10, USA.
9. Kowler, E. And Steinman, R. M. (1977). The role of small saccades in counting. Journal of Vision Research, 17, 141-146, USA.
10. Kowler, E. And Steinman, R. M. (1979). Miniature saccades: Eye movements which do not count. Journal of Vision Research, 19, 105-108, USA.
11. Kowler, E. And Steinman, R. M. (1980). Small saccades serve no useful purpose. Journal of Vision Research, 20, 273-276, USA.
12. Kowler, E., and Zingale, C. (1985). Smooth eye movements as

indicators of selective attention. In Journal of Attention and Performance XI (Eds. Posner, M. I. And Marin, O. S.M.) L. Erlbaum, Hillsdale, NJ., USA.
13. Kowler, E., Anderson, E., Dosher, B. And Blaser, E. (1995). The role of attention in the programming of saccades. Vision Research, 35, 1897-1916, USA.
14. Kowler, E., Erkelens, C.J. and Spekreijse, H. (2001) Eye Movements and Vision in the Natural World. Special issue of Journal of Vision Research, Volume 41 (Nov-Dec), USA.
15. Kowler, E., Martins, A. J., and Pavel, M. (1984). The effect of expectations on slow oculomotor control--IV: Anticipatory smooth eye movements depend on prior target motions. Journal of Vision Research, 24, 197-210, USA.
16. Kowler, E., Murphy, B. J. And Steinman, R. M. (1978). Velocity matching during the smooth pursuit of different targets on different backgrounds. Vision Research, 18, 603-605, USA.
17. Kowler, E., Pizlo, Z., Zhu, G.L., Erkelens, C., Steinman, R.M., and Collewijn, H. (1991). Coordination of head and eyes during the performance of natural (and unnatural) visual tasks. In The Head-Neck Sensory Motor System, (Edited by Berthoz, A., Graf, W., and Vidal, P.P.) Oxford University Press, N.Y., USA.
18. Kowler, E., van der Steen, J., Tamminga, E. P., and Collewijn, H. (1984). Voluntary target selection for smooth eye movements in the presence of superimposed, full-field stationary and moving stimuli, Journal of Vision Research, 24, 1789-1798, USA.
19. Mishra, S. and Satpathy, J. (2014). Reflections On Neuropsychological - Decision Making, 3rd International Conference on Managing Human Resources at the Workplace, 05 - 06 December, Mysore, India.
20. Satpathy, J and Mohapatra, B.B. (2015). Peep into Behavioural Science of Choice, International Journal on Research and Development - A Management Review (IJRDMR), Vol. 4, Issue 4, Pp: 69 - 78, ISSN: 2319 - 5479, Bhubaneswar, India.
21. Satpathy, J and Pati, P. (2016). Unmapped Territory in Neuro-decision Modeling, International Journal on Research and Development - A Management Review (IJRDMR), Vol. 5, Issue 3, Pp: 15 - 29, ISSN: 2319 - 5479, Bhubaneswar, India.
22. Satpathy, J. (2012). Neuro - Business Actors in Organisational Decision Making: An Anthology, Proceedings of National Conference on Perspectives on Employment Relations, Dated December 22 - 23, Berhampur University, India.

23. Satpathy, J. (2013). Issues in Neuro-Management Decision Making, International Journal of Business Management, Vol.2, Issue. 02, December 2012. ISSN: 2231 - 5470, India.
24. Satpathy, J. (2015). Anthology on Leadership Neuro-Decision VUCA Architecture, Proceedings of KSOM's 8th National Management Convention on The Endless Pursuit of Winning in the VUCA Environment, KIIT School of Management, January 30 - 31, 2015, Bhubaneswar, India.
25. Satpathy, J. (2015). Neuro-Based Decision-Making Challenges for Project Manager, Conference Proceedings, TECHMA 2015, Institute of Technology Management, DRDO, 26 - 27 October, Mussoorie, India.
26. Satpathy, J. (2015). Neuro-Perspective in Leadership Decision-Making Efficacy, International Journal of Multidisciplinary and Academic Research (SSIJMAR) Vol. 04, No. 03, June, (ISSN 2278 - 5973), India.
27. Satpathy, J. (2015). Random Thoughts on Leadership Behavioural Competence, Conference Proceedings, TECHMA 2015, Institute of Technology Management, DRDO, 26 - 27 October, Mussoorie, India.
28. Satpathy, J. (2015). Research Note on Cerebral - Underpinning in Neuro - Leadership Decision Modeling, Impact Factor 5. 09, ITIHAS - The Journal of Indian Management, ISSN 2249 - 7803, Vol. 5, No. IV, Oct-Dec 2015, Hyderabad, India.
29. Satpathy, J. (2016). Cerebral Underpinning in Neuro - Leadership Decision Making (Poster), neuropsychobusiness Conference, June 2-3, 2016, Bonn, Germany.
30. Satpathy, J. And Datta, T. (2014). Contributions to Neuro-Decision Computational Modeling, 41st Annual Conference of Orissa Mathematical Society and International Conference on Industrial Mathematics and Scientific Computing, No. ICIMSC14/OMS41/06, 4th and 5th January 2014, Department of Mathematics, School of Applied Sciences, KIIT University, Bhubaneswar, India.
31. Satpathy, J. And Mishra, S. (2014). Paradigm Tectonics in Neuro-Choice Making, 3rd International Conference on Managing Human Resources at the Workplace, 05 - 06 December, Mysore, India.
32. Satpathy, J., Das, A., Suneetha, N., Sturman, A. And Das, S. (2016). Crafting Neuro Business - Leadership Decisions, International Journal of Trend in Research and Development, Volume 3(5), ISSN: 2394-9333, Pp: 469 – 478, India.
33. Satpathy, J., Mishra, S. And Rath, B. P. (2014). Explorations in

Neuro-Decision Making, Odisha Journal of Social Science, Vol. I (1), Pp: 101 - 111, Odisha, India.
34. Satpathy, J., Mohapatra, B.B. and Sturman, M. (2015). Leadership Neuro-Choice Mechanism, International Journal on Research and Development: A Management Review (IJRDMR), Volume: 4 Issue: 1, ISSN (Print): 2321- 5747, Bhubaneswar, India.
35. Tiwari, P., Satpathy, J. And Mishra, S. (2014). Cerebral 'Paths' in Techno-Leadership Continuum: Some Human Resource Perspectives, Proceedings of UGC - Sponsored National Seminar on Management Practices and Sustainable Development, 23 - 24 March, F M University, Balasore, Odisha, India.

CHAPTER 2

EMERGING TECHNOLOGIES IN HEALTHCARE POST-COVID ERA

S. GEETHA PRIYA[1], ASHISH BHATTARAI[2], AISHWARYA SWAIN[2], SHREENANDAN SAHU[2], RAVI KANT AVVARI[2*]

[1]Department of Biotechnology, Sri Shakthi Institute of Engineering and Technology, Coimbatore – 641062, Tamil Nadu, India
[2]Department of Biotechnology and Medical Engineering, National Institute of Technology Rourkela, Odisha – 769 008, India

ABSTRACT

The COVID-19 pandemic has caused a rapid decline in the world's economic growth by rendering many people jobless. During the pandemic, the management of critical patients in Intensive Care Units (ICUs) was the major challenge faced by healthcare professionals. Recently contactless or contact-free services have brought a lot of opportunities in the healthcare industry post-pandemic period, which includes telemedicine, telecommuting and mobile transactions. As direct person-to-person contact is avoided, people's purchasing behaviours have also seen a lot of transition. Thus, the pandemic has accelerated the digitalisation of various medical applications, including self-diagnosis app services, digital tracking of confirmed cases, etc. As far as recent developments in medical device development are concerned, advanced information technology has paved the way for more innovative design, as in the utility of artificial intelligence (AI), Internet of Things (IoTs), 3D Printing, Smart Sensors, and Drones, which have been instrumental in providing contactless services. Despite these advancements, the challenges faced by the medical device manufacturing industry are regulatory complications, high healthcare costs, and slow, expensive R&D.

Keywords: *COVID-19; Smart Sensors; Telemedicine; Internet of Things; Communication Technologies; Artificial Intelligence*

1. INTRODUCTION

One of the deadliest issues in the world today, the 2019 coronavirus disease pandemic, has claimed many lives. The virus that causes coronavirus disease is contagious and spreads from infected people through airborne droplets.

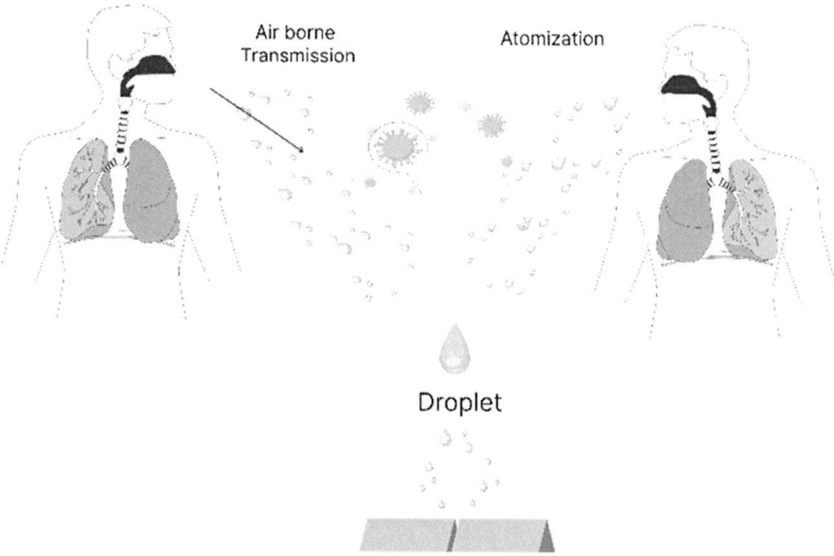

Fig. 1: Transmission of the viral particles through air/ contact media

The main symptoms of this disease include fever, headache, cough, nausea, vomiting, fatigue and breathlessness. One of the main methods currently available to detect the virus is real-time Reverse Transcription Polymerase Chain Reaction (rRT-PCR). After the onset of this disease, several vaccines have been developed, approved and sent to various countries for the mass vaccination campaign. Other ways by which we can minimise the spread of this disease are by wearing masks in public places, social distancing, quarantining, frequently washing hands and proper ventilation of indoor spaces. In addition, the government has taken many steps to minimise the spread of the disease by restricting the population in crowded and busy places like schools, colleges, companies, industries, hospitals, banks, buses and trains, malls, movie theatres, shopping markets etc. As a result, the COVID-19 pandemic has decreased the economic growth of countries worldwide. This has rendered many people jobless across the world. Furthermore, as the pandemic is highly contagious, it was challenging for the healthcare professionals like clinicians to treat patients infected with this disease. This has been even more cumbersome if the patients are in severe conditions, especially in Intensive Care Units (ICU), as close monitoring of the patients is required.

2. STANDARD OPERATING PROCEDURES PRE/ POST COVID

Standard operating procedure (SOP) is a set of written instructions that describes the step-by-step process, such as storing records, screening and enrolling subjects, collecting data and submitting Institutional Review Board (IRB) applications and their renewals that must be taken to perform the routine activity properly. In the context of COVID-19, it describes the detailed process of managing discarded potential COVID-19 vials and associated activities. It also provides clear instructions on the appropriate treatment to minimise any associated health risk considering the local context.

Table 1: COVID-19 risk indicator

Alert Level	Disease situation	Health care system	Disease control	Community measures
Level 1 Normal	Cases and outbreaks have been reported.	No infections among healthcare workers	Completely quarantine contacts and isolate cases	Schools begin with safety precautions—large-scale events with security measures. Businesses implement safety measures such as distancing, disinfection, and so on.
Level 2 Low Risk	Spreading less widely Rear outbreak	Capable of safely dealing with cases of rare infections	Greater capacity to quarantine contacts and isolate cases	Businesses and schools open with safety precautions like hand sanitiser and distancing; no vulnerable staff or students; some mid-size mass gatherings with safety precautions; and healthcare facilities with safety precautions.

Level 3: Moderate Risk	lessening of the spread and few outbreaks	Some capacity to safely care for cases.	Some ability to isolate cases and quarantine contacts	Keep your outside travel to a minimum. school closures and e-learning; fewer small mass gatherings; Safety precautions taken by businesses; Altered health care services
Level 4: High Risk	Several outbreaks	Limited capacity to safely care for cases	Limited or no ability to isolate cases and quarantine contacts	Stay at home; School closures and online learning; No mass gatherings; Essential services only; Modified health care services

Testing standards during the Covid phase

The virus that causes COVID-19 is examined by testing specimens from the respiratory tract of infected individuals' noses or mouth areas. Nucleic acid amplification tests (NAATs) and antigen testing are the primary categories of viral diagnostics. Depending on the testing technique's availability and the patient's severity, one test type may sometimes be advised over another. NAATs are a particular PCR-based test often carried out in a lab. Antigen tests are quick tests, giving findings in 15 to 30 minutes. However, further NAAT may sometimes be advised to validate the results of an antigen test.

Quarantine – Different levels

Quarantine is the restriction of movement or activity of people who are healthy but may have been exposed to infection to prevent the spread of infectious diseases and illnesses. This includes sealing regional or local borders and constructing a cordon sanitaire – a physical barrier around a specific area to forbid entry and exit. According to the information that is currently available, a quarantine period of 14 days is the most effective way to reduce the chances of spreading a contagious virus or disease. However, while quarantines are an essential tool in helping to reduce the spread of infectious diseases, they do not guarantee complete protection against infection. These are the many levels of quarantine which are:

Enhanced community quarantine (ECQ)

- First implemented on March 17, 2020
- Regardless of age or health, there is no movement

- There is no economic activity except for utility services, food, water, and other essential sectors.
- No public transport and physical classes

Modified enhanced community quarantine (MECQ)

- First implemented on May 16, 2020
- Limited movement of people to get essential services and to go to work
- As the economy slowly improves, only a few factories and processing plants can run at total capacity.
- Limited access to critical goods and services when it comes to transportation
- Limited transportation for those going to work and for essential services and classes is suspended at all levels.

General community quarantine (GCQ)

- First implemented on May 1, 2020
- There will be little movement, but the government and almost all industries—aside from those involving large crowds of people—will be permitted to operate up to 75% of their capacity.
- Limited transportation options with social distancing
- Face-to-face instruction is not allowed, but flexible learning is permitted.

Modified general community quarantine (MGCQ)

- First implemented on May 16, 2020
- Permissible socioeconomic activities that adhere to the bare minimum of public health requirements

SOP Implementation Problems During COVID-19

Most medication research, testing, manufacturing, and marketing programmes have standard operating procedures (SOPs), and they understand the significance of these procedures. However, there needs to be better knowledge of many aspects of standard operating procedure (SOP) design, maintenance, training, and organisation. This lack of understanding results in stacks of issues with regulatory compliance, which are found during FDA audits. Because of this, pharma businesses and their workers, who rely on SOPs to guarantee that safe drugs are created, tested, manufactured, and sold, might run into a significant amount of trouble. This article discusses some of the most frequent problems that arise during the development, administration, and execution of SOPs. Some of the reasons causing issues in the implementation of SOP are:

a) Inadequate SOPs

Many regulations require the creation of standard operating procedures (SOPs). The guidelines made available by the FDA, ISO, and ICH frequently cover requirements for standard operating procedures (SOPs). For organisations to satisfy these preconditions, SOPs need to be developed to guarantee quality uniformity and conformity with relevant industry regulations. Extensive explanations of the criteria can be found in several chapters and parts of Title 21 of the Code of Federal Regulations. These explanations are cited in their entirety below (CFR). To ensure that the clinical laboratories can carry out their day-to-day operations in a manner that is both quality-conscious and compliant, they must develop standard operating procedures, also known as SOPs.

b) Lack of proper maintenance of SOPs

Time and experience both contribute to the evolution of procedures. However, due to the absence of formal definitions for updating SOPs in a written document, most of the healthcare industry still needs to formalise the procedural changes that have been incorporated into their most recent version of their SOPs. As health parameters and laws change with time, it is necessary to revise any previously written standard operating procedures (SOPs) currently in place to account for how time and conditions have shifted. The healthcare industry should implement a policy that requires SOPs to be reviewed and updated regularly to keep up with the ever-changing times and circumstances. It is of the utmost importance to keep detailed records of the procedures followed when updating previously established SOPs, developing new ones, and training, retraining, and authorising staff in all processes. The presence of written and formalised procedures helps ensure that employees are appropriately trained in their roles, reducing the likelihood that mistakes or misunderstandings will occur.

c) Lack of substantial SOP training

If employees are given sufficient training, having well-written standard operating procedures (SOPs) will help them a little. The management is obligated to guarantee that all people relevant to the SOPs for which they are accountable read and comprehend those SOPs. Proper training of the operator is an essential thing to consider when new technologies emerge in the medical area. This is one of the most important things to consider. Management and the related biomedical department must design training programmes for employees and offer frequent updates to guarantee that workers are taught and aware of the SOPs. The majority of auditors have a strong interest in vital training records. They also test an employee's comprehension of the procedures by asking them to describe what is included in the SOPs and demonstrate how the work is carried out.

d) Impracticality and Owner's Objection

When developing SOPs, one must carefully define every facet of the governing processes and policies. Incorrect references, places that need to be prepared, and other such things may bring the work activities to a standstill, which will eventually hinder performance. Standard operating procedures are frequently drafted in a manner that appears impossible to execute. This will result in a chaotic jumble that needs to be better organised and will not produce the desired goals. It is also the job of the leader of the healthcare organisation to look out for the safety of the SOP's management, technical team, and security personnel. If the hospital personnel are allowed enough leeway, it will slow down the progress and provide later outcomes. In addition, the heads can raise objections to the design of the SOP if they believe it does not maximise their potential. As a result, the standard operating procedure should be created and constructed while considering the scope, budget, cost, time, and quality.

3. EMERGING TRENDS IN MEDICAL DEVICES POST COVID

The global healthcare industry has experienced rapid growth due to the COVID-19 acute emergency alarm and the subsequent pandemic phase, which forced a complete revision of the original medical equipment and diagnostic formulation idea. This update and improvement in various areas have significantly changed the methods used by engineers and medical experts. The pre-existing medical instrumentation and diagnosis techniques, such as magnetic resonance imaging (MRI), computed tomography (CT) scans, and laboratory testing, were essential in providing timely insights into patient health. Below is a list of scenarios for some of the post-COVID sectors that have undergone remodelling

3.1. Healthcare Industry Automation

The post-COVID phase of the Meditech industry presents an unprecedented opportunity to develop new solutions and technologies that focus on automating medical device production. During COVID-19, the world faced shortages of PPE, putting more pressure on manufacturing and making these available to all in a brief period.

3.2. Domestic manufacturing of medical devices

COVID-19's disruption of global supply chains has resulted in well-publicised problems with the availability of essential items such as medical supplies and protective equipment, including shortages of necessary medical equipment. The demand for medical devices has proven to be far greater than what domestic manufacturers can supply. This is because many supply chains have been set up in other countries for a long time and are heavily dependent on imports, and depending only on imports of crucial medical devices poses a significant threat to public health security. Not only does domestic production of necessary medical devices circumvent trade restrictions, but it also guarantees product quality and market stability can connect through the IoT.

3.3. Clinical trials

The most significant impact of COVID-19 on the industry was in the field of clinical trials. Many medical devices with a certain level of risk, such as implantable devices, require clinical investigations. Due to difficulties posed by travel bans, hospital/clinic visitation restrictions, and social distancing precautions, access to clinicians and patients essentially ended, and most trials were postponed or cancelled. It is necessary to alter clinical trials to remove apparent immediate risks to participants, such as switching from in-person to virtual visits, getting rid of study procedures that don't affect the validity of the research or participant safety, and adding screening questions to find potential COVID-19 exposure. Milestones may be impacted because overburdened clinical sites and healthcare professionals might have little to no interest in maintaining clinical routines and trial schedules. Unless these new medical devices are used to contain COVID-19, delays will likely affect the entirety of pipelines and product launches for large medical device manufacturers managing diverse product lines.

3.4. In silico medicine

Designing, testing, and validating medical devices using computer modelling and simulations are known as "in silico medicine," which offers enormous potential for the medical industry. In silico medicine's "AI platform" main area can quickly provide revolutionary breakthrough medications to patients while lowering costs and raising success rates. It paved the way for reinforcement learning and generative adversarial networks (GANs) to create novel molecular structures for diseases with and without known targets. Medical researchers analyse the effectiveness and safety of the device in various clinical scenarios utilising virtual human populations rather than actual human subjects or animals. For instance, a realistic lung model could be used to check the performance and safety of a ventilator design. Similarly, a virtual patient model with variable blood glucose levels might be used to verify an insulin pump with glucose monitoring. Thus, in silico medicine enables businesses to cut back on the time and expense spent on R&D while enhancing their products' quality, effectiveness, and safety. In their most recent strategic policy roadmaps and regulations, the European Union and FDA mentioned the significance of in silico medicine.

3.5. Digital twins

Digital twins are virtual representations of patients or medical equipment in the healthcare industry with prior maintenance and diagnostic information in a single knowledge base. Precision medicine, clinical trials, and public health can all benefit from its ground-breaking applications since it can simulate random perturbations on the digital twin to understand the expected behaviour of the physical twin. The associated digital twin is updated to track a patient's health more accurately as new data becomes available, such as when a patient goes to the hospital for a check-up or a medical gadget is examined. This current data can then be included in the simulation and AI models to predict future states and aid in decision-making. Patients can benefit from individualised medication by using digital twins in medical care. By using digital twins in medical care, patients can take advantage of personalised medicine to find the best treatment for themselves and take a more proactive approach to managing their chronic illnesses and general health. Digital twins allow for better product lifecycle management and predictive maintenance for manufacturers of medical devices.

3.6. Drones

Unmanned aerial vehicles, also known as drones, can be helpful for various tasks, including search and rescue operations in the aftermath of natural disasters, filming and photography in high-risk locations, and product delivery in environments where it would be risky to send human delivery personnel. Since the COVID-19 pandemic, drones have been used to collect lab samples, deliver vaccinations, medications, and medical supplies to people living in remote rural areas far from a hospital, and stop the spread of potentially fatal infectious diseases. It would be risky to send human delivery personnel. Disinfectant is frequently sprayed by drones into public areas to clean up polluted sites. Drones are commonly used for this purpose. One more use for communication drones is in the medical field, specifically for diagnosing, treating, evaluating, and monitoring patients in remote areas. The use of drones could also be beneficial for patients who are unable to prepare their meals due to medical issues. These drones could bring them food and other necessities, eliminating the need for carers to travel while exposing themselves to the risk of contracting an infection.

3.7. Augmented reality and robotics

To help surgeons prepare for their next jobs, virtual reality and augmented reality (AR) technologies are being employed in classrooms. Particularly in surgical training, these technologies allow trainees to practise in a simulated environment to improve their skills while minimising patient risk. Employing AR might result in significant resource savings. To simulate a real surgical or operating procedure, for instance, you would put on a pair of glasses to see the wound in three dimensions. This would save you from bringing in a large operating table and contaminated body parts. In addition to protecting hospital money, this can add interest to training. This will allow medical personnel to receive training on any technique and keep up with new developments in the field. According to "The American Nurses Foundation," 52% of U.S. nurses have considered leaving their professions due to severe workloads. Robots can be utilised to help medical professionals care for patients more effectively while reducing the overall stress of the hospital's workforce. The usage of hospital robots for many functions, such as patient monitoring, defibrillator use, streamlining clinical workflow, transporting hospital resources, etc.

4. TELEMEDICINE, TELECOMMUTING AND MOBILE TRANSACTIONS

The pandemic has seen a dramatic rise of the popularity in the usage of mobile devices. Contract-free services such as telemedicine gained more acceptance in this situation, where video or phone consultations can be used to allow for accessible communication between the patient and the doctor. Most medical professionals prefer to view their patients on laptops or smartphones. Health organisations provide their clients with virtual appointments and are growing their telehealth offerings. Telemedicine has become simpler thanks to recent technological advancements. Through the mobile app, patients use telemedicine and seek virtual consultations with medical professionals. Telemedicine or telehealth is helpful in many aspects, especially regarding comfort and convenience. When patients are ill, they do not need to wait in long lines at the doctor's office. Even with a busy schedule on both ends, it also saves time. Telemedicine, often known as telehealth, also stops the spread of infectious diseases. Patients are pre-screened for potential infectious diseases during telehealth consultations.

Tele medicine

The pandemic's problems have been addressed with remote care through telehealth, home monitoring, and self-administered care; these methods won't go away when the threat is finally eliminated. Utilising digital information and communication technologies, telehealth, and remote monitoring allow you to access healthcare services from a distance and manage your health. For instance, video can be used in place of, after, or in addition to a face-to-face appointment with a doctor. It is common to practise administering remote care using telemedicine tools, especially in the United States, where 63% of healthcare professionals did so during the COVID-19 outbreak. One of the main themes in response to the COVID-19 epidemic has been the ability of digital technology to keep people connected despite physical distance, facilitating the development of remote monitoring devices. In addition, home monitoring systems and self-administered care have been used to support those affected by the pandemic, allowing people to take control of their health with heart rate monitors, blood pressure monitors, and other connected medical devices.

Telecommuting

Telecommuting is how one works from home using email, the Internet and the telephone. This is mainly done to minimise the spread of infectious and contagious diseases. Telecommuting is advantageous in many ways. For example, it reduces the expenses of employees, promotes work-life balance and increases flexibility. However, there are some limitations associated with telecommuting, such as less personal contact with co-workers and hindered communication. Moreover, it will be more difficult for the supervisors to monitor the employees from their homes. As a result, there may be decreased productivity.

Mobile Transactions

Mobile transactions have increasingly become popular post-COVID-19. As many people have been immobilised due to the pandemic, people could not move from their residences to ATMs and banks to purchase household items. As a result, people have started using mobile transactions, which are more convenient, safe and secure. Another advantage of using mobile transactions instead of using cards or cash payment is that it is less likely to be lost or stolen.

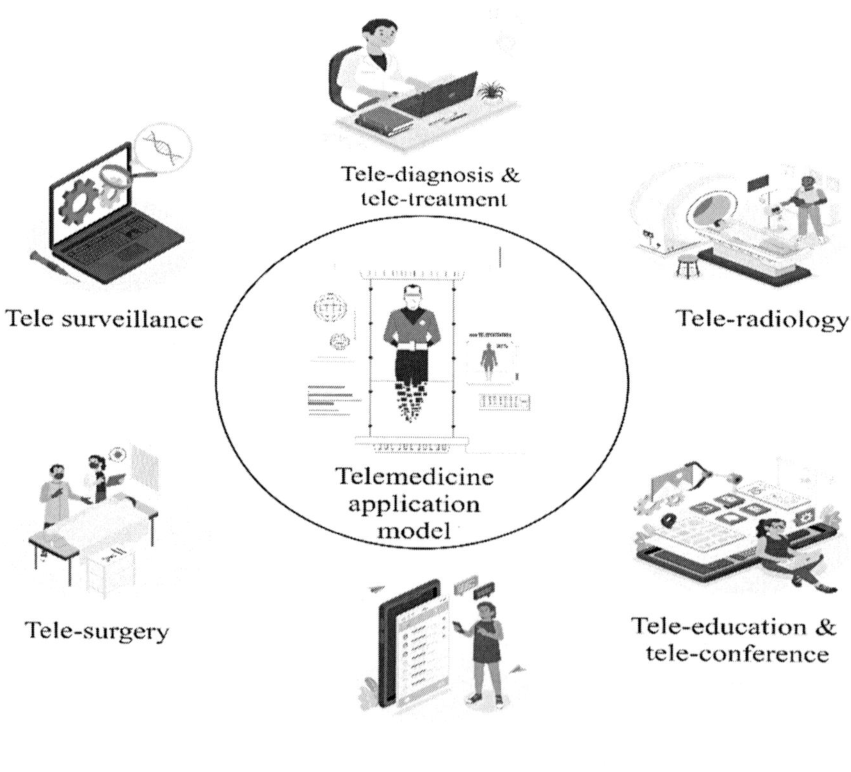

5. 3D PRINTING

Building a three-dimensional object from a computer-aided design (CAD) model or adding consecutive layers of material while a computer controls the design model are two examples of various applications that may be accomplished using three-dimensional (3D) printing. Generating complicated items with variable geometries, which are difficult to construct by hand, is one of the primary advantages of three-dimensional printing (3D printing). CAD software allows defects in a model to be located and fixed before it is printed, resulting in fewer errors overall. The Society of Manufacturing Engineers published Rapid Prototyping and Manufacturing: Fundamentals of Stereolithography under the ISBN. It is anticipated that most future uses of 3D printing technology will be found in dentistry and hearing aids. Using 3D bioprinting technology by several biotechnology companies for tissue engineering has made it possible to create organs and other body parts using inkjet printing techniques. This has been made possible as a result of the advancements that have been made in the field of tissue engineering. Cells are placed onto a gel matrix using this technique, and the structure, including the vasculature, is gradually built up over time. In response to the COVID-19 pandemic, several pieces of protective gear, such as face shield frames, have been printed using 3D printers. When there was an outbreak of COVID-19, 3D printers were used to make essential supplies.

6. ARTIFICIAL INTELLIGENCE IN BIOMEDICAL DEVICE DEVELOPMENT

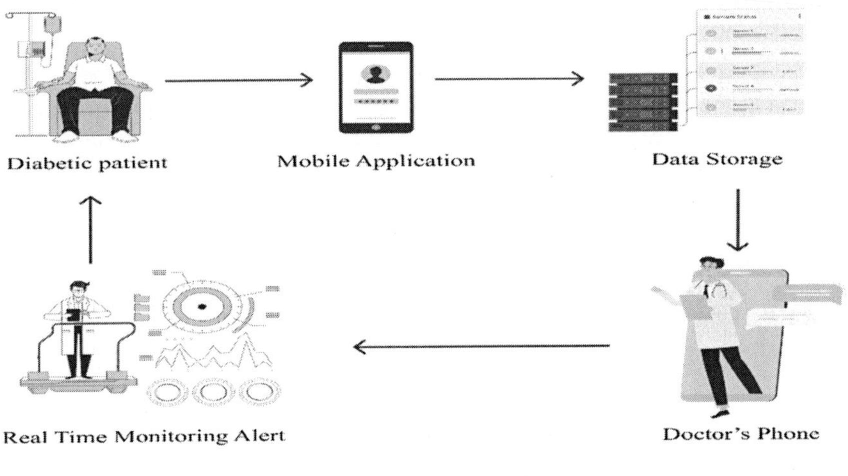

Artificial intelligence is one of the most potent technologies known to improve capabilities in all aspects of industries. Artificial intelligence in healthcare technologies has indeed revolutionised the healthcare industry. It has helped many healthcare practitioners worldwide to diagnose and treat diseases effectively. The technology that mimics human activity, learning and decision-making is known as artificial intelligence. AI-based devices can automatically evaluate a large amount of data from multiple sources and pinpoint the trends for monitoring and predicting which patients have an increased risk of disease so that the treatment can be done effectively based on the medical records. AI-based devices serve three main essential functions the Internet of Things (IoT), Medical Imaging and Chronic Disease Management. IoT uses wireless and digital services to manage patient data and monitor patients more effectively and efficiently with reduced costs.

Medical imaging companies reduce a patient's exposure to radiation by providing better image quality and clarity. In chronic disease management, artificial intelligence incorporated into medical devices can treat patients by providing proper medication. For example, in the case of people affected by diabetes, the patients can wear biosensors that monitor blood sugar levels and administer insulin at regular intervals. Additionally, IoT can reduce medical costs significantly by reducing the number of medical tests and visits required for diagnosis.

7. DISCUSSION AND CONCLUSION

After the COVID-19 era, the development of medical devices has undergone a significant amount of digitalisation. This digitalisation began with telemedicine, a practice in which patients and medical professionals interact with one another by scheduling appointments over the phone or via video call. As the pandemic continued to deteriorate for a considerable amount of time, it gave rise to a phenomenon known as "telecommuting," in which employees work from home by communicating through the phone, email, and the Internet. The workers have reported significantly less stress, pressure, and financial strain due to this, and they have also reported increased flexibility in their working hours. In addition, due to the pandemic, more people are turning to mobile transactions rather than paying with cash or credit cards to reduce the risk of spreading the disease. Additionally, there has been an increase in the use of artificial intelligence in the development of biomedical devices, particularly in

- the Internet of Things is characterised by the utilisation of digital and wireless services for managing patient data.
- Medical imaging improves diagnostic clarity while lowering a patient's exposure to potentially harmful radiation.
- Managing patients' chronic diseases ensures they have access to the appropriate medication.

New technologies have led to the implementation of three-dimensional printing, which can be used in conjunction with computational tools and three-dimensional printers to produce three-dimensional objects such as face shields. In addition, during a pandemic, unmanned aerial vehicles, also known as drones, have collected lab samples and transported vaccines to remote areas to stop the spread of infectious diseases that can cause severe or even fatal illnesses.

CHAPTER 3

IMPACT OF THE COVID-19 PANDEMIC ON MEDICAL DEVICES IN HEALTHCARE

AISHWARYA SWAIN, ASHISH BHATTARAI, SHREENANDAN SAHU, RAVI KANT AVVARI

Department of Biotechnology and Medical Engineering, National Institute of Technology Rourkela, Odisha – 769 008, India

ABSTRACT

The healthcare industry, in particular, has experienced ups and downs during the COVID-19 crisis, whether for prevention, diagnosis, or therapy. Where the pandemic has driven us to look for opportunities under necessity, this chapter gives a broad overview of the COVID-19 scenario in healthcare services concerning healthcare solutions. The chapter discusses delays in non-emergency medical procedures, amendments in rules and regulations during the pandemic, use of medical devices and diagnostic products, protective devices for prevention and imaging modalities and sensors for COVID-19.

Keywords: *COVID-19; Healthcare; Medical Devices*

1. INTRODUCTION

"*In crises, it is acceptable to have more questions than answers. There's no room for 'not invented here' in a crisis. In a crisis, we should all be learners.*" These recent past years of the COVID phases of the COVID-19 pandemic have revealed vulnerabilities in the medical field, resulting in our health system's actual visuality. Even the developed countries, which tend to show their superiority, have gone through dark phases of the pandemic. How much stronger is the government, either by leadership, economic influence, political influence, or strong international and military alliances? If the health economy followed by proper health education is not sound to every resident, the nation's overall strength drags down.

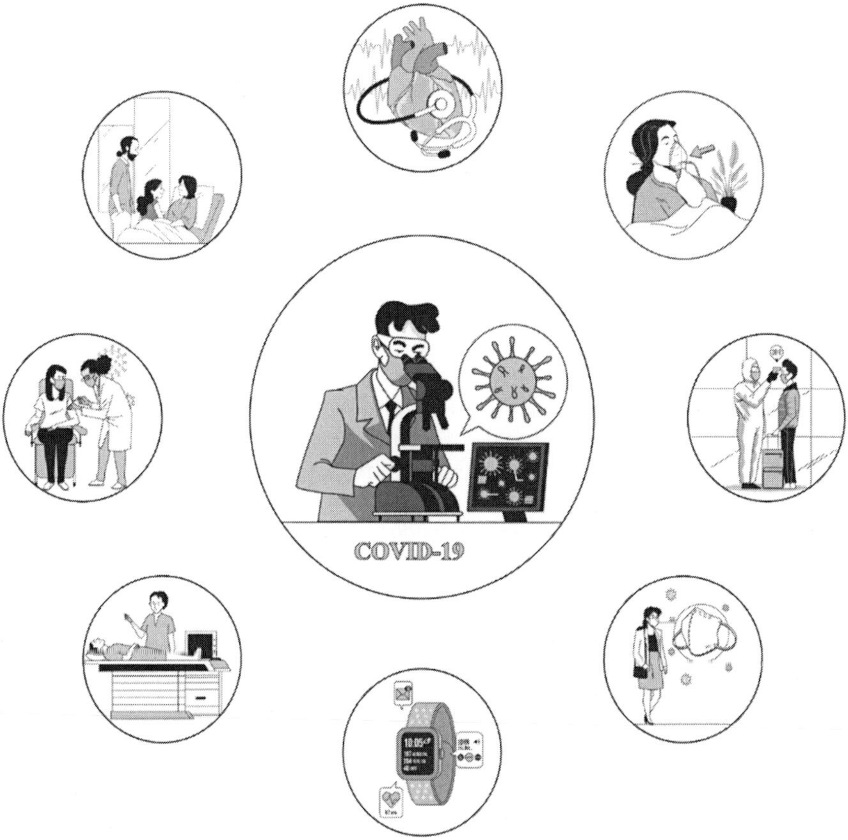

Fig. 1: COVID-19 scenario in healthcare services

The healthcare industry, in particular, has experienced ups and downs during the COVID-19 crisis, whether for prevention, diagnosis, or therapy. Broadly, the health industry has become concentrated on the medical device industry with peerless demand for some critical products such as diagnostic kits, ventilators, and personal protective equipment (PPE).

Manufacturers highly focused on medical devices were significantly affected during the pandemic, especially from March to April 2020, which are considered to be non-essential or non-urgent. Although within a particular month, nearly all markets engaged in medical devices gained momentum from the significant dip in sales caused by COVID-19 until the second wave was detected. The Alpha variant, first documented in the UK, which was rapidly spreading around the globe for months finally, leads up to its peak in January 2021. Again, the next massive wave caused by the Delta variant peaked between the summer and fall of 2021 and has again disrupted the usual supply chain of medical devices.

2. TEMPORARILY SHUTDOWN & DELAY OF NON-EMERGENCY MEDICAL PROCEDURES

However, all medical devices are not essential in the management of patients during the pandemic. *Per se*, there was a drastic drop in elective medical procedures or non-emergency medical procedures, and among those, many of which were postponed or cancelled to free up beds after the exponential growth of patients affected by COVID, which resulted in a shortage of medical assistance. This allowed hospitals to focus more on treating COVID-19 patients, thereby minimising patient time and preventing/taking preventive measures from spreading in the hospital setting. Some of these medical procedures were temporarily delayed, as discussed in the following.

Aortic and coronary stent grafts: Aortic and coronary stent grafts alike are minimally invasive as there is a requirement for the insertion of a small tube into the aorta or coronary artery to effectively hold the blood vessel open and prevent it from closing and blocking the channel. Following the procedure, since the patients have to stay at the hospital for recovery and under supervision, there is an increased chance of patients being infected by the virus.

Aesthetic procedure: Cosmetic surgeries involving breast implantation, Lipoplasty and non-essential dental practices have been delayed due to the pandemic. Such practices were postponed further as it does not come under the emergency category.

NTDs – Neglected Tropical Diseases: More than 20 common illnesses fall under the category of NTDs. These diseases impact more than one billion people and are responsible for 500,000 deaths annually. The great majority of these deaths occur in Africa, Asia, and the Americas. Because diagnostic technologies are readily available, the number of initiatives that aim to control or eradicate NTDs has increased. For instance, owing to the availability of RDTs to map the spread of the illness and effective treatments to treat it, the Global Lymphocytic Filariasis Eradication Program (GPELF) is regarded as one of the most successful public health projects. Its goal is to eradicate the disease. Let's compare the NTDs programme to the COVID pandemic. The number of diagnostic tests that have been created for COVID in the last few years is comparable to the number of diagnostic tests that have been generated for NTDs over the past hundred years. However, the catastrophic effects of COVID-19 have diminished both the planned results and the progress that has been made. It is possible that decreased financing, human resources, clinical trials, and field deployment may put NTD diagnostics in a precarious position, particularly concerning their research and development requirements.

Orthopaedic surgery: Orthopedic patient care has been significantly disrupted. The backlog of surgeries and outpatient visits has yet to be fully recovered, which could lead to a significant deficit by the end of 2020. While increased use of satellite practices appears to continue in 2022, annual surgeries were further reduced.

2. AMENDMENT IN RULES AND REGULATIONS IN THE FIELD OF GLOBAL HEALTH ADMINISTRATION

An emergency use authorisation (EUA) was implemented by the Food and Drug Administration (FDA) in response to the declaration that COVID-19 constituted a public health emergency. A EUA is granted during times of crisis when there are no adequate, approved, or otherwise readily available alternatives, which can lead to a delay in the delivery of potential aid and an increased mortality rate. Several businesses in the healthcare industry that had previously acquired FDA clearance from the United States for their diagnostic tests have expanded production to assist with the current testing shortage. They can also accelerate pre-market studies, enabling products to be brought to market more swiftly. The revised International Health Regulations (IHR) provide a legal framework to address the issues of disease prevention and detection via global surveillance and reporting system. The framework has set minimum mandatory controls at the national level to prevent disease. These regulations aim to frame reasonable laws at the global level to control infectious diseases. Unfortunately, the IHR could only be applied to a few specific disorders. There were only three of them (cholera, plague, and yellow fever). It needed an epidemic of a new coronavirus for international action to be taken, even though appeals had been made for the IHR to be revised. The update to the IHR that took place in 2005 offers the current legal framework that may be used to identify, prevent, and react to international public health crises. In response to healthcare emergencies, the World Health Organization (WHO) has invoked the "*Public Health Emergency of International Concern*" (PHEIC) declaration six times to control the international spread of infectious diseases. These diseases include polio, Zika, influenza H1N1, and Ebola, including the recent COVID-19.

3. GLOBAL SCENARIO ON MEDICAL DEVICES DURING COVID-19

One of the majorly changed areas for most MEDTECH companies was the impact on their sales force and service teams of medical devices or the raw material mainly required for the manufacturing of medical devices. Both of these factors were interrupted as many countries went into a lockdown state, leading to travel restrictions that hampered the flow of devices and services across borders. Also, post-sales activities, including installation and maintenance, had become very difficult to carry out. Some examples of majorly impacted medical equipment are described below:

In vitro diagnostic products: There was an increase in the demand for diagnostic testing to perform preliminary viral infection testing and assess the disease's spread. Following this emergency, several biotechnology, pharmaceutical, and medical device companies started shifting their operations to an *in vitro* diagnostic (IVD) production pipeline. This led to more emphasis on the development of point-of-care devices. The PCR (polymerase chain reaction) assay tests are the most common type of these testing kits. The test requires collecting a swab sample from the patient's mouth or nose and identifying the genetic code for SARS-CoV-2 in those who are already infected with the virus.

Ventilators: Patients who have been infected with COVID-19 require ventilator support to breathe and have any chance of making a full recovery. Before the pandemic, the healthcare system did not have sufficient ventilators to treat patients who needed them. However, sudden increases in demand lead the industry to develop innovative new ways to produce quick, affordable, and reliable ventilators.

Table 1: List of medical devices and their usage during COVID-19

Sl. No.	Device Name	Purpose	Utility of the device
1.	Ventilator a. Intensive care b. Transportable c. Anaesthetic ventilator	Used to pump air into the lungs that help an individual to breathe, by which respiratory failure can be avoided.	Frequent
2.	Filters for ventilator		
3.	Extracorporeal membrane oxygenation (ECMO), equipment and disposables	It is similar to a heart-lung bypass machine mainly used for children in COVID time in the intensive care unit.	Frequent
4.	Colourimetric end-tidal CO2 detector	They are used to get thorough information on the adequacy of circulation in the lungs.	Frequent
5.	Oxygen delivery devices like a. Oxygen masks b. Venturi masks c. Oxygen tents d. Oxygen head boxes e. Bag valve masks f. Flow-splitter g. Oxygen Humidifier	It draws in air from your surroundings, removes nitrogen and other gasses and delivers pure oxygen to the patient.	Frequent
6.	Medical gas cylinder	Gases like oxygen, nitrous oxide, medical air, Entonox, carbon dioxide and heliox are stored and supplied as required.	Frequent

7.	Endotracheal intubation devices and kits	For endotracheal intubation, reach out to the trachea for possible oxygenation/ delivery of medicine.	Moderate
8.	Nasopharyngeal airway devices	It is a soft rubber tube that assists with patient oxygenation and ventilation, which have difficulty oxygenating or ventilating via bag-mask ventilation.	Frequent
9.	Needles, catheters, cannulae, connectors, oxygenators, and tubing	For intravenous fluid delivery and drug administration.	Moderate
10.	Syringe pumps	To administer a minimal amount of medication or any fluid into the patient's body.	Moderate
11.	Disposable emergency cricothyrotomy set	With significant aerosolisation during COVID-19, there is an increased risk for infection. The set allows for airway for ventilation and passage of Oxygen.	Frequent
12.	Fiberscopes	They are used to study and analyse difficult-to-reach parts of the human body. It is used for diagnosis during COVID.	Moderate
13.	Blood Pressure monitoring kits	It is used to measure the blood pressure of an individual, which helps in the self-health monitoring of COVID patients during a pandemic.	Frequent
14.	Computed tomography (CT) scanners	Used to confirm the PCR diagnostic test and false CXRs results during COVID and mainly chest CT is used.	Frequent
15.	Ultrasound machine	It is a simple, fast and portable imaging solution when scanning for COVID-19.	Frequent
16.	Electrocardiograph	It is a simple, non-invasive bedside tool that is extremely useful and gives an early diagnosis and treatment of cardiac injuries to COVID patients.	Frequent
17.	Manual resuscitator	A type of manual ventilator is provided to COVID patients facing problems with breathing.	Moderate

18.	Dialysis machine and bloodlines, including CRRT machines	They are used to treat COVID patients with kidney injuries.	Frequent
19.	Pulse oximeter	For measuring the oxygen saturation level and monitoring the health of the patient	Frequent
20.	Thermometers	For measuring the temperature of patients suffering from fever, as in COVID-19	Frequent
21.	Blood gas syringes	To monitor the arterial *blood gas* (ABG) and acid-base patterns *in COVID-19*	Frequent
22.	Medical drills for vascular access	To access vascular for dialysis	Moderate
23.	Hemofiltration equipment	We used hemofiltration therapy to replace kidney function in acute renal failure with COVID-19 infection.	Moderate
24.	Anti-decubitus mattress	They were used for bedridden COVID patients to prevent bed sores.	Moderate
25.	Suction devices	Used to ventilate COVID patients	Frequent
26.	COVID-19 Test Kit a. PCR b. Antigen c. Inflammation tests	Used to screen subjects with the infection	Frequent

Personal protective equipment (PPE)

In response to the sanitation guidelines issued by the WHO and the demand from healthcare professionals treating infected patients, a variety of personal protective equipment (PPE) such as sanitisers, medical masks, gloves, and ventilators are being pulled from the shelves of their storage facilities. It is implemented to safeguard workers in situations where engineering and administrative controls cannot be reasonably expected to bring hazards down to tolerable levels. When it comes to the personal protective equipment industry, most nations are highly dependent on the medical components produced in China, which is one of the leading exporters of PPE on a worldwide scale. Most governments have prohibited the export of medical parts and equipment to deal with spiking demands during the pandemic. In doing so, these countries have put themselves in danger of violating the fundamental premise underlying the GATT 1947 agreement. This has resulted in significant disruptions to supply chains in the personal protective equipment (PPE) sector across nations highly dependent on medical imports.

Identifying the type of personal protective equipment (PPE) necessary based on the results of a danger assessment might be helpful. Many different kinds of safety equipment may be used in the workplace, and the one that should be used is determined by the present hazards and the working circumstances. The following are essential PPE that can help protect a medical person from the COVID environment:

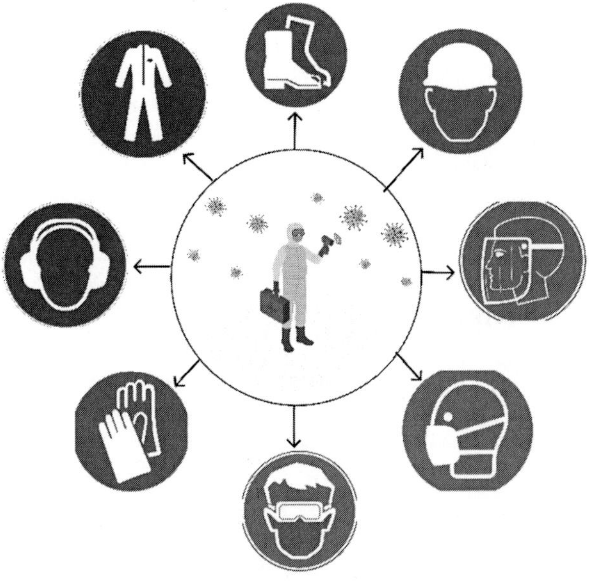

Fig. 2: Variety of personal protective equipment for protection from COVID-19

Respiratory Protective Equipment: RPE protects users from inhaling harmful substances that may cause pathological conditions. Toxic gases, dust, powders, chemicals, and splatter may contain COVID-19-causing bacteria and viruses. Healthcare workers and industrial workers wear RPE in hazardous environments. Respiratory protective equipment prevents the inhalation of harmful substances that can cause a variety of pathologies. Toxic gases, chemicals, and splatter may contain COVID-19 and other viruses and bacteria. In addition, these materials have COVID-19-contaminated splatter. Healthcare workers, industrial workers, firefighters, and others who work in hazardous environments wear PPE. There are two main types of Respiratory Protective Equipment listed below:

- **Respirators / Filtering devices** – They use filters to purify the air before it is breathed in by removing contaminants from it. **Example: Half masks, Full face masks, Powered**
- **Breathing apparatus** – Supplies clean air from an independent source to the wearer before direct inhalation. Example: Fresh air hose, Constant air hose, Demand valve

Skin and Body Protection: Another type of PPE is classified as "skin" and "whole body" protection, where it includes a wide range of safety footwear, gauntlets, armlets, body protection, coveralls, etc. The skin's surface may become contaminated by various chemicals and dangerous pathogenic environments while directly infecting the person. All kinds of chemicals and hazardous pathogenic environments may cause contamination of the skin's surface while directly infecting the individual.

- **Body protection:** *Overalls, Aprons, Harnesses, Life jackets.*
- **Hand and arm protection:** *Gloves, Wrist cuff armlets*
- **Foot protection:** *Safety boots, Wellington boots, Anti-static footwear*

Eye protection: Protection for the eyes PPE is primarily used for activities that risk causing eye damage or loss of vision, as well as burns, splashes, and sprays of toxic liquids. As a result of working in an environment with a high incidence of contagious diseases, the risk of contracting the virus through one's eyes must be seriously considered. As such, it is critical to ensure that all workers are provided with adequate eye protection through safety glasses, goggles, or face shields to prevent the spread of infection, which follows the ANSI Z87.1 eye protection standard. ***Example: Safety glasses, Face shield, Splash goggles.***

Hearing Protection: Hearing protection equipment (HPE), also known as personal protective equipment (PPE) for hearing, is required to be worn by workers to protect their hearing. This is accomplished by reducing the amount of noise energy and other disease-causing pathogens that enter the inner ear and cause damage to the ear. As a result, PPE for hearing is essential to minimise the potential damage caused by noise and pathogen exposure. It is crucial to have a clear idea of how you intend to use HPE so you can select the appropriate device for your needs. HPE is available in various forms, dimensions, and degrees of safety, so it is essential to choose the suitable device as per need. ***Example: Ear plugs, Ear muffs, Semi inserts***

Vaccine kits: COVID-19 vaccinations are available and on their way throughout the world. The world now faces a massive logistical challenge: maintaining these vaccines in the ideal storage conditions to guarantee the stability and efficacy of each dosage administered. Because some of these vaccines must be kept frozen or chilled for maximum safety and efficacy, this is an even more complicated issue. While giving vaccines at neighbourhood drug stores, community centres, or clinics has been successful in many US communities, there are still numerous locations both inside and outside the country where these cold-storage systems fall short. Many middle- and low-income nations lack sufficient storage facilities. The difficulty of maintaining freezing temperatures is significantly more incredible in warmer regions, such as South America, Asia, and Africa, especially in isolated settlements or places without electricity. This implies that they have few COVID-19 vaccination alternatives.

Inventory risk is the first. Increased inventory reduces the return on capital if vaccinations are produced but not sold. The second difficulty is getting credit. A company could not have the working capital to purchase inputs even though it has a legally enforceable commitment. Giving the money up ahead can solve this issue with advance purchases. The identification and removal of supply bottlenecks represent the third problem. Once vaccine manufacturers have made purchases, they can then make purchases from suppliers, and so forth. Several governments have signed options contracts or memorandums of understanding without a legally enforceable promise to buy. These contracts do not solve the problem.

4. ROLE OF IMAGING MODALITIES AND SENSORS FOR COVID-19

Technological progress has been a recurring concern for humanity in recent decades. Technology companies offer many innovations to address common healthcare care problems. For example, the coronavirus has taken hold of Earth and is being combated through digital interventions across affected geographic boundaries and territories.

In a radiographic examination of COVID-19, imaging modalities such as Chest Radiography (CXR) have been employed to study the changes in the anatomical structures of the chest in patients infected with the virus. Studies show the early course of the developed may also be possible to detect even before the development of the symptoms in the patient. Positive radiographs of the lung show fuzzy patches on the bilateral surface of the lung, the location and severity of which change with the stage of infection. The lung opacities increase in texture, firmness, and seriousness as COVID-19 inflammation progresses in the affected lungs. The COVID-19 CXR findings become apparent 10-12 days after the initial onset of the disease. COVID-19 CXR findings share considerable similarities with viral pneumonia. Therefore, radiologists are challenged in the differential diagnosis of COVID-19 compared with viral pneumonia. Other modality includes ultrasound, computed tomography, magnetic resonance imaging and positron emission tomography.

While the above imaging technique involves a heavy machine fixed at a location, the mobile ultrasound is challenging to use as a temporary measure for patient diagnosis at an isolated place. Therefore, there is a need for an intelligent sensing health monitoring system that caters to the immediate screening of the subjects. During the COVID phase, it was challenging to undergo standard medical health check-ups due to various restrictions so that IoT-based arrangements can be beneficial to individuals for routine health check-ups. COVID-19 patients must be regularly informed about their health conditions, particularly their body temperature, heart rate, and oxygen saturation (SpO2). This particular system makes use of a total of six sensors to collect data from the hospital environment. Some primary sensors are as follows: a heartbeat sensor, a body temperature sensor, a room temperature sensor, a CO sensor, an O_2 sensor, and a CO_2 sensor.

In contrast to conventional imaging modalities, electronic sensors have been very useful in measuring health parameters relevant to patient monitoring. In times of physical distancing, sensors allowed for remote monitoring of the patients as well as diagnosis. For example, a heartbeat sensor is instrumental in assessing heart function. The plethysmography theory serves as the basis for constructing the heartbeat sensor that was later developed. It achieves this by measuring the change in blood volume that takes place via any individual's organ due to the light-intensity movement through that organ. This may be done to anybody. However, timing is of the utmost significance when it comes to devices designed to monitor the heart's pulse rate. This is because the heart beats at a constant pace. The speed at which the heart beats controls how the blood is distributed throughout the body, and the signal pulses created when the blood absorbs light is analogous to the signal produced by the heartbeat. The pulse oximeter is also used to measure the subject's oxygen saturation levels (SpO2), which typically lie in the range from 95 to 100%. However, with COVID-19, the oxygen saturation levels drop below 95%, causing depletion in Oxygen and leading to shortness of breath and hypoxia.

Alongside the developments during the pandemic, body temperature measurement has its significance in screening and monitoring subjects. Body temperature is a vital indicator of the fever resulting from infection. Body temperature can be readily measured using an onboard temperature sensor such as using LM35 Sensor, which is an accurate temperature sensor whose output voltage is directly connected to the temperature in centigrade, and the temperature may be stated in either degrees Fahrenheit or degrees Celsius. In addition, technologies using infrared sensing have been prevalent in screening the subject without having direct contact with the skin. IR thermometers and thermal imagers provide a quick view of the body temperature as a point measurement or thermal image. By following the temperature variation, real-time assessment of the body temperature can be made with possible diagnosis at an early stage and detection of any fever symptoms during treatment.

Assessment of heart function is equally essential for the subject. With the pandemic, there has been increased emphasis on remote monitoring, which has led to the adoption of wearables for remote sensing. In contrast to the conventional ECG, where the gels are applied to increase the effective contract with the skin, dry electrodes are potentially helpful in developing wearable ECG, with promise for long-term heart monitoring.

Likewise, monitoring of the ventilation is also essential. With the assistance of these oxygen sensors, which may also be integrated into ventilators, it is possible to estimate the percentage of oxygen present in the gas mixes used for breathing. The Oxygen Sensor monitors are included in a re-measure gas monitor (RGM), the quantity of oxygen present in a gas mixture, in addition to the particular cells. Oxygen sensors are sometimes referred to as FiO2 sensors, and one of the names for these sensors is O2 Cells. The quantity of oxygen present in the gas mixture is referred to as the fraction of inspired oxygen (FiO2) in the scientific community. The oxygen content of room air can be deduced from the fact that the gas mixture that constitutes atmospheric room air contains a proportion of inspired oxygen equal to 21% and that the concentration of oxygen in room air is also similar to 21%.

CONCLUSION

The COVID-19 pandemic has reshaped the medical device market with a core focus on making the services available during the pandemic through innovation and the use of digital technologies. From regulation to policy changes, the pandemic has taught us new ways to deal with the situation while ensuring diagnosis and monitoring through innovation in medical devices.

CHAPTER 4

THE VIROLOGY OF THE COVID-19 PANDEMIC: UNDERSTANDING A GLOBAL HEALTH CRISIS

PRIYA CHOUDHARY, ANUSHKA SAMANT, SAURABH KUMAR GUPTA, SIRSENDU SEKHAR RAY

Department of Biotechnology and Medical Engineering, National Institute of Technology, Rourkela 769 008, Odisha, India

ABSTRACT

In addition, to bringing about influenza or pneumonia in individuals, coronaviruses (CoVs) also cause an extensive range of illnesses in domestic and wild animals, fowl, and rodents, counting slight to severe abdominal, respiratory, and systemic sicknesses. HCoV 229E, NL63, HKU1, and OC43 cause cold symptoms in immunocompetent persons. The zoonotic coronaviruses SARS-CoV and MERS-CoV can cause deadly respiratory illnesses. The national authorities in China informed WHO on December 31 that there were patients with pneumonia of unclear aetiology. The coronavirus reading group designated this virus as severe acute respiratory syndrome coronavirus 2 (SARS-CoV-2) and coronavirus disease 19 for the current outbreak of a coronavirus-associated acute respiratory sickness (COVID-19). The first instances of COVID-19 were discovered in Turkey on March 10, 2020, and after one month, there were 47,029 cases and 1006 fatalities. As of 10 April 2020, 1,727,602 confirmed SARS-CoV-2 cases had been reported in additional than 210 countries, with 105,728 fatalities.

Keywords: *Human Coronaviruses: HCoV, Middle East corona virus: MERS- CoV, animal coronaviruses, history of coronaviruses, COVID-19, SARS-CoV-2*

1. INTRODUCTION

"The planet requires immense positive energy to combat negative forces. Go to the core of your inner self and generate positive energy for the sake of humanity." A virus is an infectious agent composed of nucleic acid segments (DNA or RNA) encased in a protein coat. A virus must infect cells and use host cell machinery to replicate. Viruses are unable to reproduce on their own. The host cell may die as a result of the viral infection process. HIV, measles, smallpox, and coronaviruses are well-known for their capacity to infect humans with sickness. The SARS-CoV-2 epidemic two years ago caused a global pandemic that disseminated coronavirus illnesses (also known as "COVID-19") among people. We have learned much more about viruses over the last two years. People can contract viruses. But in reality, a vast range of creatures are infected by viruses. Certain viruses, for example, can also be infectious to bacteria and fungi. We could learn much about how viruses survive by studying the viruses that infect such a diverse range of organisms. This truly aids our understanding of how diseases affect people. However, only a small percentage of viruses cause human disease. The most abundant viruses, often known as phage, are the ones that infect bacteria most frequently. They are substantially more abundant even though they have many of the same traits. Future research will focus on the mechanisms by which viruses infect people and any potential strategies for preventing viral replication in human cells. The SARS-CoV-2 virus causes infectious condition known as COVID-19, or coronavirus disease. Shown in Figure (1).

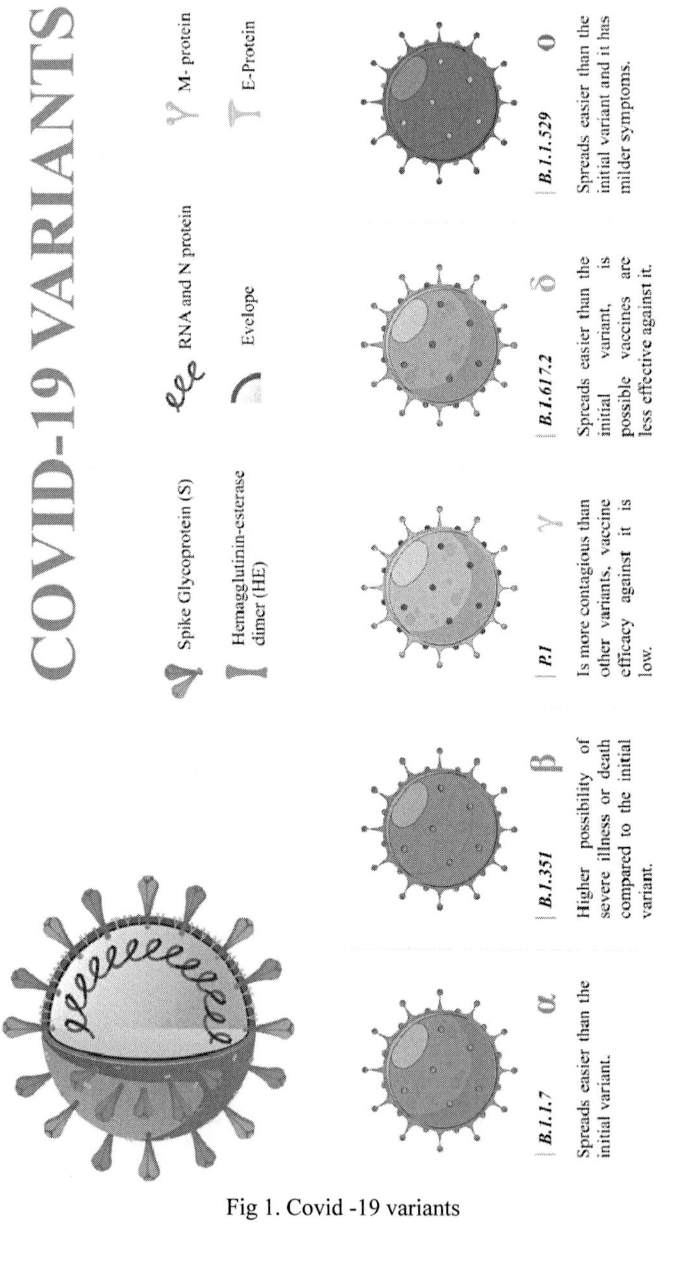

Fig 1. Covid -19 variants

2. BACKGROUND OF CORONAVIRUS

IBV, found by Beaudette & Hudson in sick chickens with respiratory difficulties, was the first coronavirus (1937). The murine and hepatitis viruses (MHV) were discovered in 1949 by Cheever et al. First reported in 1946, swine-transmittable gastroenteritis. In 1965, Tyrrell and Bynoe discovered the first human coronavirus in a schoolboy's cold-infected trachea organ culture (B814). Under a microscope, the virus resembles avian IBV. Procknow and Hamre detected five viral strains in tissue cultures from sick medical students. Almeida and Tyrrell compared the morphology of the HCoV 229E prototype strain to B814 and IBV. HCoV OC43, the prototype strain, and three other strains believed to be immunologically different to OC43 or 229E were among the six additional strains found utilising organ culture.

In 2002–2003, Guangdong, China, saw unusual and deadly pneumonia. This sickness became severe acute respiratory syndrome (SARS). The virus spread quickly via international air travel, generating outbreaks in Vietnam, Singapore, Canada, and others. Hong Kong's first case was in late February. 916 (10.8%) of the 8422 patients reported from 29 countries on six continents in July 2003 died. In response to the demand for exotic food, Guangdong's live animal marketplaces keep, exchange, and provide restaurants with a variety of animals. SARS-animal CoV's reservoir debut occurred then. Small mammals traded in these markets, such as civet cats, have been shown to carry viruses linked to the SARS-CoV, making it likely that these marketplaces were the first to transmit the virus to humans. The first MERS-CoV isolate was identified in the lungs of a 60-year-old Saudi patient with severe pneumonia and renal failure. Live MERS-Coronavirus, which is identical to the virus seen in people, was identified from dromedary camel nasal swabs, confirming that camels are reservoir hosts. MERS-CoV is one of the deadliest viruses ever identified in humans, with nearly 2500 laboratory-confirmed cases as of February 14, 2020, and a 34.4% case fatality rate.

3. HISTORY OF COVID-19

A 41-year-old man was hospitalised at Wuhan's Central Hospital six days after the disease started on December 26, 2019. He had a fever, tightness in the chest, dry cough, and weakness for a week while not having diabetes, hepatitis, or tuberculosis. The patient worked at a neighbouring indoor fish market that sold hedgehogs, badgers, snakes, and birds, both live and dead. After an epidemiological examination, the Wuhan Centre for Disease Control and Prevention found that the patient had no memory of handling live poultry, and no bats were being sold. China reported 44 cases of pneumonia without a known cause to WHO between December 31 and January 3, 2020. During the reporting period, no accountable agent was found. The National Health Commission of China provided WHO with new information concerning the outbreak's link to a Wuhan City seafood market on January 11 and 12. The Chinese discovered a new coronavirus variety on January 7, 2020, allowing other countries to create specialised testing equipment. China revealed genetic information on the coronavirus on January 12, 2020. The Thai Public Health Ministry reported the first imported case of the (2019-nCoV) novel coronavirus from Wuhan, Hubei Province, China (January 13, 2020). On January 15, 2020, Japan's Ministry of Health, Labour, and Welfare confirmed an imported case of 2019-nCoV from the same source (MHLW). The Democracy of Korea's National IHR Focal Point (NFP) proclaimed Wuhan, China's first case of a novel coronavirus on January 20, 2020. COVID-19 first appeared in Turkey on March 10, 2020. 47,029 cases and 1006 deaths followed one month later, as of April 10, 2020, 1,727,602 SARS-CoV-2 infections in over 210 countries had resulted in 105,728 deaths. SARS-CoV-2 infections are already frequent.

4. SEVERE ACUTE RESPIRATORY SYNDROME CORONAVIRUS-2

According to phylogenetic analysis, the 2015 bat SARS-like coronavirus sequence was significantly clustered with the 2019 nCoV, and structural analysis revealed changes to the spike glycoprotein and nucleocapsid protein (previously known as SARS-CoV-2). As a result, the 2019 nCoV is distinct from SARS, which bats presumably spread before undergoing a mutation that allowed it to infect people. The Coronavirus Study Group officially designated this virus as severe acute respiratory syndrome coronavirus two based on the phylogenetic tree, taxonomy, and established practises (SARS-CoV-2). Coronavirus Disease-19 is the name of the current outbreak of acute respiratory sickness caused by a coronavirus (COVID-19).

5. WHAT IS THE ORIGIN OF CORONAVIRUSES?

Typically, camels, cats, and bats are hosts to coronaviruses. Although viruses exist in animals, they do not infect them. On rare occasions, a variety of animal species can become infected by these viruses. Viral transmission may lead to virus evolution (mutation). Eventually, the virus could migrate from animal populations to human populations. It is thought that the first infections with SARS-CoV-19 occurred at a grocery store that sold live animals, seafood, and meat.

6. HOW MAY ONE OBTAIN COVID-19?

SARS-CoV-2, also known as COVID-19, can enter the body through the mouth, nose, or eyes. After that, it makes its way to the mucous membrane located at the back of your throat and the rear of your nasal passages. After it has attached itself to those cells, it will begin to proliferate to prepare for its invasion of the lung tissue. It is possible for the virus to then travel to other tissues of the body from there.

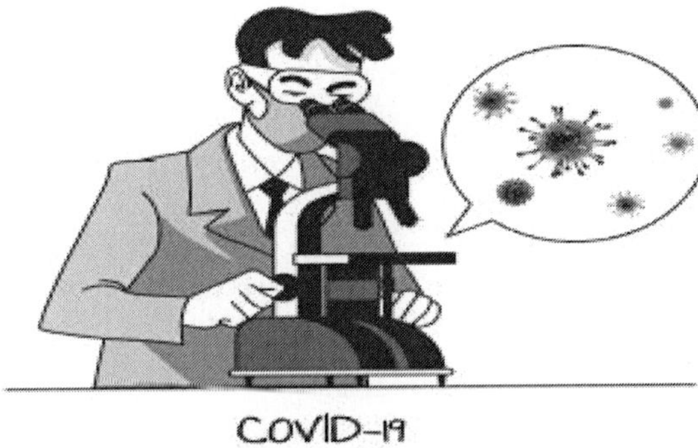

Fig 2. COVID-19: A major threat.

7. FOR HOW LONG MAY SOMEONE BE INFECTED WITH THE COVID-19 VIRUS?

It may take a few days after being infected with COVID-19 before you start showing symptoms, but you will remain contagious until your condition improves. If you've had symptoms for ten days after they first appeared, you're no longer contagious.

8. WHO IS MOST SUSCEPTIBLE TO COVID-19?

The likelihood of contracting COVID-19 is higher for those in the following groups: How soon after contracting SARS-CoV-2 will I start to exhibit COVID-19 symptoms? Between contracting the virus and showing symptoms is the incubation period, which can span two to fourteen days. It typically takes five days for symptoms to appear. The severity of the symptoms might range from quite mild to very severe. Though this may alter as variations appear, only moderate symptoms affect about 80% of COVID-19 individuals.

9. CAN ONE CONTRACT COVID-19 AGAIN IF ONE GET'S WELL AFTER HAVING IT ONCE?

Before, it was thought that three months must have elapsed since your prior positive test if you have become re-infected with SARS-CoV-2. SARS-CoV-2 reinfection before the omicron version was infrequent but possible. Astronomers discovered Omicron (B.1.1.529) in November 2021, and it quickly spread to other parts of the world. Omicron's numerous alterations allowed it to attack the immune systems, so we had more reinfections than ever before. The COVID-19 virus is still capable of reinfection since it is constantly changing. The immunisation regimen, including a booster dosage, is the best defence against serious illness.

10. CAUSES AND SYMPTOMS

Various individuals exhibit various COVID-19 symptoms. In reality, a few infected individuals display no sickness symptoms (asymptomatic). However, the following indications and symptoms are regularly mentioned by those who have COVID-19:

- Cough, cold or fever.
- Trouble breathing or shortness of breath.
- Tiredness.
- Body aches or muscle pain.
- Headaches.
- New odour or taste loss.
- Throat pain
- Runny nose or congestion
- Vomiting or nauseous.
- Diarrhoea.
- There may be more symptoms.

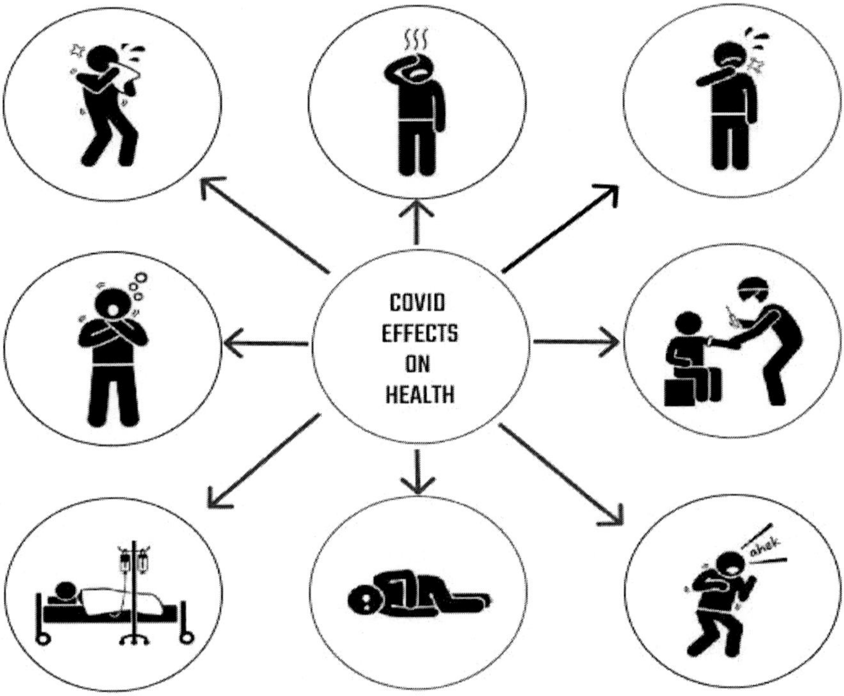

Fig 3. Covid -19 symptoms: Effect on health

It could take anywhere from two to fourteen days for symptoms to present once the virus has been injected. Children's symptoms are comparable to those of adults, albeit typically in a more moderate version. People over the age of 65 and those who already have major underlying medical disorders are more prone to experience more severe COVID-19 problems.

11. HOW CAN I AVOID ACQUIRING COVID-19?

Getting vaccinated is your most effective method of protection against COVID-19. One should take the same precautions to avoid catching them as one would to avoid catching other viruses like the flu or the common cold. This is the best way to avoid catching them. You should wash your hands for at least 15 seconds every time you wipe your nose, use the restroom, or come into touch with someone contagious. This includes before and after you use the restroom. As directed by the Centre for Disease Control and Prevention (CDC), outfit your face with a multilayered, cloth facemask that provides a snug fit and covers your lips, nose, and chin.

If you want to keep infections from spreading from your hands to other parts of your body, you should avoid touching your nose, eyes and mouth. When you cough or sneeze, cover your mouth and nose with a tissue or cough into your sleeve to prevent germs from spreading. Throw away the tissue. It would help if you properly washed your hands after that. Never cough or sneeze into your hands! Maintain a 6-foot minimum separation from somebody who is contagious (6 feet is ideal). Keep to your home while you are ill.

Keep your distance from large groups of people if you have a compromised immune system or a history of sickness and have been advised to do so. It is especially important during outbreaks for you to pay close attention to the advice that is offered by the healthcare authorities in your area. To sanitise frequently touched surfaces and eliminate viruses, apply a disinfectant (such as doorknobs and countertops). If you do not have soap, you should use a hand sanitiser which contains at least 60 per cent alcohol. Ensure you get adequate sleep, stick to a nutritious diet, drink lots of water, and get some form of physical activity whenever possible. Your immune system will be strengthened, and you will be better able to defend yourself against illnesses if you do these things.

It was the first serious illness to emerge in the new millennium that spread rapidly and showed a blatant aptitude for doing so along international air travel routes. It was also the first disease that spread quickly. Anything that a sick person has touched has the potential to spread SARS to others indirectly. SARS patients were mostly healthy 25-70-year-olds. However, SARS may have affected some under-15s. SARS-like infections kill 3% of sufferers. Most infected patients recover without specialised care from moderate to severe respiratory infections. However, some people get serious illnesses that require medical attention.

Older adults and those with pre-existing conditions like cancer, diabetes, chronic lung disease, or cardiovascular disease are more prone to get serious illnesses. COVID-19 can kill anyone, regardless of age. Understanding the disease and how it spreads is the best method to prevent and reduce transmission. Keep at least one metre between you and others, wear a mask that fits, and periodically wash or give your hands an alcohol-based hand massage to prevent infection. When it is your turn, you should receive your immunisation, and you should pay close attention to any local information that is provided to you.

12. EVOLUTION OF THE COVID 19 VIRUS

When cases of pneumonia with no apparent explanation started to appear in Wuhan, China, scientists immediately realised that a new strain of the SARS-CoV had appeared. The Wuhan Huanan Seafood Wholesale Market was linked to the earliest cases during the first few weeks of the epidemic in Wuhan (which will be referred to in the following paragraphs as the "Huanan market"). The great majority of the reported occurrences involved market vendors and active dealers. The Wuhan Huanan Seafood Wholesale Market had to close while conditions were at their worst. The government banned the sale of environmental disinfection and sanitisation products on January 1st, 2020. The market, which mostly sold seafood and aquatic products and other goods created from domesticated and wild animals, was initially thought to be the pandemic's epicentre. This gave birth to the hypothesis that an error in human-animal interaction caused the pandemic. However, investigations conducted in the past revealed that there were more people with an illness that started in December 2019. Furthermore, not all of the early cases indicated a link to the Huanan Market. It has not been demonstrated via subsequent epidemiological or epizootic research that COVID-19 can be transmitted from civets or pangolins to humans. This is true even though it was first thought that pangolins and civets might have been to blame for the COVID-19 pandemic and the severe acute respiratory syndrome epidemic between 2002 and 2004. (SARS).

The identity of the likely intermediate host for the SARS-CoV2 infection is uncertain. It has been discovered that a variety of significant zoonotic viruses, including the Nipah, Hendra, and SARS-CoV viruses, as well as coronaviruses with significant genetic diversity, are transmitted to people through bats. It is particularly important to take into account the coronaviruses associated with the human SARS and Middle East respiratory disease (MERS) epidemics in 2002 and 2013, respectively, when discussing COVID-19. The virus that was determined to cause COVID-19 was quickly isolated from patients and sequenced; the outcomes from China were then shared and reported in January 2020. According to the research, it was a brand-new positive-stranded RNA virus from the Coronaviridae family (a subgroup B betacoronavirus).

The virus had never before been observed in humans. Early research indicated a startling similarity between the genetic sequence of the new virus (SARS-CoV-2), which triggered SARS in the years from 2002 to 2004, and the coronavirus that caused SARS during those years (SARS-CoV) (another subgroup B betacoronavirus). The following year, a substantial quantity of research on sequencing and phylogeny was conducted worldwide. The results of the effort have been shared all around the world and are being archived on the GISAID platform. The RaTG13 coronavirus strain and SARS-CoV-2 are nearly identical, sharing 96.2% of the same amino acid sequences. A sample from a horseshoe bat was previously sent for genetic sequencing (Rhinolophus species) to identify this strain.

Additionally, there are some minor similarities between SARS-CoV-2 and a pangolin strain. RaTG13 is the name given to the viral segment most closely resembles the SARS-CoV-2 segment. SARS-CoV2, like SARS and MERS coronaviruses, spread swiftly amongst humans. However, the virus was more infectious than these two coronaviruses. SARS-CoV-2 exhibits broad tissue tropism due to the spike protein's affinity for ACE2 (ACE2). Respiratory viruses seldom infect blood vessel endothelial cells. The virus also causes hypercoagulability, strong immunological responses from multiple organs, and long-term effects. Viruses caused these traits. Even before symptoms appeared, SARS-CoV-2 carriers were contagious. Infections can cause nothing, mild disease, serious illness, or death. Infections cause several diseases. The joint WHO-China mission on COVID-19 was established in February 2020 to educate planners in China and around the world about the next steps in the epidemic response.

This expedition collected planning data. Its goals include: to better understand the COVID-19 outbreak as it spreads in China, as well as the nature and results of current containment measures; to promote information sharing about the COVID-19 response and preparedness measures being implemented in nations that have been affected by or are at risk of importations; to develop recommendations for altering COVID-19 containment and response measures in China and internationally; and, finally, to better understand The OIE, FAO, and countries have been asked to "continue to work closely with countries to identify the zoonotic source of the virus and the route of introduction to the human population, including the possible role of intermediate hosts, including through efforts like scientific research" as part of the One-Health Approach. In July 2020, the WHO referred a team to China to decide how to find the virus's origin. The seventy-third World Health Assembly suggested this. The Terms of

Reference defined the investigation's scope, guiding principles, and expected conclusions. These Terms of Reference need two phases of research: Phase 1 would investigate how the virus moved to Wuhan, while Phase 2 would expand on the discoveries and scientific literature (Phase 2). The Terms of Reference required a global collaborative team of specialists to support and conduct Phase 2 studies and analyse Phase 1 outcomes and design. The experiment would help us comprehend the virus's origins. The study's findings and generalisations will improve global readiness for SARS-CoV-2 and other similar zoonotic viruses.

13. EPIDEMIOLOGY

Before the joint investigation, COVID-19 is thought to have first surfaced in Wuhan around the start of December 2019. According to preliminary data from severe pneumonia surveillance, there had not been any obvious clustering or deviance from patterns in the months and weeks before the initial cases of the illness were reported. Since many people with SARS-CoV-2 infection are symptomless or only experience mild symptoms, there may have been additional infections when the initial cases were identified, and transmission may have occurred in the population earlier. Therefore, it is essential to investigate the likelihood of past events happening again. The Huanan market, where people could buy animals and animal products, was linked to several early cases. It was uncertain if the market caused the virus's first human encounter or aggravated the outbreak. Early on, the Huanan market was said to be unrelated to Wuhan's other markets. This market may have propagated SARSCoV-2, according to some studies. Many Phase 1 investigations were chosen after the ToRs were created in July 2020, and work was completed before the international team arrived in January 2021. Data collection, purification, clinical record review, patient interviews and testing, and preliminary research were needed for this project. Based on their findings, the WHO and Chinese teams performed more studies. Before the outbreak was officially declared in Wuhan in December 2019, the studies used monotonous disease and death monitoring data, medical histories, and targeted SARS-CoV-2 laboratory testing to establish if Wuhan or Hubei Province had SARS-CoV-2 transmission. After confirming the outburst, they sought transmission in Wuhan and Hubei Province. Both goals had to be achieved.

14. SARS-COV-2 VARIANT TRACING

SARS-CoV-2 evolves like many viruses. Most changes don't influence the virus's properties. However, the virus's propagation, the severity of sickness, and other factors may affect the efficacy of immunisations, medicinal medications, diagnostic technology, and other public health and social activities. Since January 2020, WHO has monitored and analysed the virus's progress with associates, expert linkages, national establishments, institutions, and academics to predict SARS-expected CoV-2's future. In the latter part of the year, the World Health Organization (WHO) and its global networks of experts are monitoring the virus to ensure that, if significant amino acid substitutions are found, we can inform nations and the public about any potential adjustments that may be needed to respond to the different and stop its feast. Global methods are being developed to detect "signals" of probable volatile organic compounds (VOCs) or volatile organic contaminants (VOIs) and assess their public health risks. National authorities may categorise local issues according to their choices. Preventing introductions into animal populations and reducing disease transmission through tried-and-true processes and disease management are the two most critical parts of the global effort to decrease mutations that harm public health. WHO-recommended therapies and precautions stop new viral strains. Public health and social programmes (PHSM), particularly IPC programmes, reduce COVID-19 instances, hospitalisations, and deaths in areas with high VOC transmission rates. National and local governments should expand PHSM and IPC activities. Authorities should also increase surveillance and sequencing capabilities and employ a rigorous approach to examine SARS-CoV-2 variant transmission in the local environment and identify anomalous epidemiological occurrences. This prevents SARS-CoV-2 strains from spreading.

15. NAMING VARIANTS OF SARS-COV-2

To name the SARS-CoV-2 genetic pedigree, scientists have been using the nomenclature systems from GISAID, Nextstrain, and Pango. Nextstrain, Pango, and GISAID are the firms that created these systems. To discuss labels that are simple to pronounce and do not stigmatise VOI and VOC, The WHO Virus Evolution Working Group, WHO COVID-19 reference laboratory network, GISAID, Nextstrain, and Pango, and other virology, microbial nomenclature, and communication professionals from numerous nations and agencies met. This event's goal was to encourage public discussion on Greek Alphabet letters. The WHO-convened expert committee has lately recommended them because they are simpler and more useful for communicating these concepts to non-scientific audiences. The term "index virus" should be used when employing this naming technique and referring to the SARS-CoV-2 genome sequence discovered in the initial instances (December 2019). These operational definitions of SARS-CoV-2 may need to be modified more frequently in the future as the virus that origins SARS-CoV-2 is always evolving, and our knowledge of the consequences of the virus's different strains is constantly growing. When appropriate, variations may be categorised as VOCs, VOIs, or VUMs, even if they match all the requirements for these classifications. The Technical Advisory Group on Virus Evolution may also classify low-threat variants as essential (the Virus Evolution Working Group).

16. CONCERNING THE VARIOUS VARIATIONS (VOC)

Definition in operation:

SARS-CoV-2 variant that fits the requirements for the VOI is connected to one or several of the modifications listed below to a significant extent important to global public health, including A rise in disease transmissibility or a downward trend in the SARS-CoV-2 epidemiology; OR, an increase in the disease's virulence or a change in how the disease manifests clinically; OR, a decline in the efficacy of available diagnostics, vaccines, or treatments; OR, an increase in the disease's virulence.

17. VARIANTS OF INTEREST (VOI)

Operational definition SARS-CoV-2 substitutes have the following traits:

- Possessing genetic alterations that have been predicted to affect, or are known to affect virus features like transmissibility, diagnostic or therapeutic escape, the severity of the illness, immunological escape; and
- Recognised as a source of considerable community transmission, several COVID-19 hotspots in many nations, with a growing comparative prevalence and caseload over time, or other obvious epidemiological impacts pointing to a rising threat to global public health. However, there isn't currently a popular kind that is of interest (VOI).

18. VARIANTS UNDER MONITORING (VUM)

Working definition: Although there is no firm proof of the influence of genetic alterations on a SARS-CoV-2 variant, the alterations are suspected to modify virus characteristics on phenotypic or epidemiological outcomes at this time, additional surveillance and repeat assessment are required in the absence of new data. The WHO designations will not yet be offered because of the possibility that our understanding of these variants' impacts could change fast and that designated variants under monitoring could be added or removed without much difficulty. However, under this heading, past VOIs/VOCs may be observed for a considerable amount of time and will keep the WHO categorisation they were given until further notice.

19. EPIDEMIOLOGICAL UPDATE ON COVID-19 (2019-2022)

Over 114,000 deaths and roughly 20 million new cases were reported globally from January 2 to January 29, 2023; these figures represent drops of 78% and 65%, respectively, from the previous 28 days (Figure 1, Table 1). Recently, the Western Pacific region has seen an upsurge in cases and fatalities, particularly in China, which has dominated epidemiologic trends. As of January 29th, 2023, more than 6.8 million fatalities and over 753 million confirmed cases were registered worldwide. Prevalence studies have shown that the current trends in reported COVID-19 cases underestimate the number of infections and reinfections worldwide. The drop in testing and the backlog of reports in many countries are some of the causes of this. This report may contain only some of the necessary information. Therefore, it should be interpreted carefully.

Additionally, information from previous weeks is regularly updated to reflect adjustments made by governments to their previously reported COVID-19 cases and fatalities. We will now show changes in epidemiological trends over four weeks. This evens out the weekly variations in case counts and gives a more accurate depiction of where the cases are speeding or receding. Weekly statistics are still available on the WHO COVID-19 dashboard, where you can download the whole report.

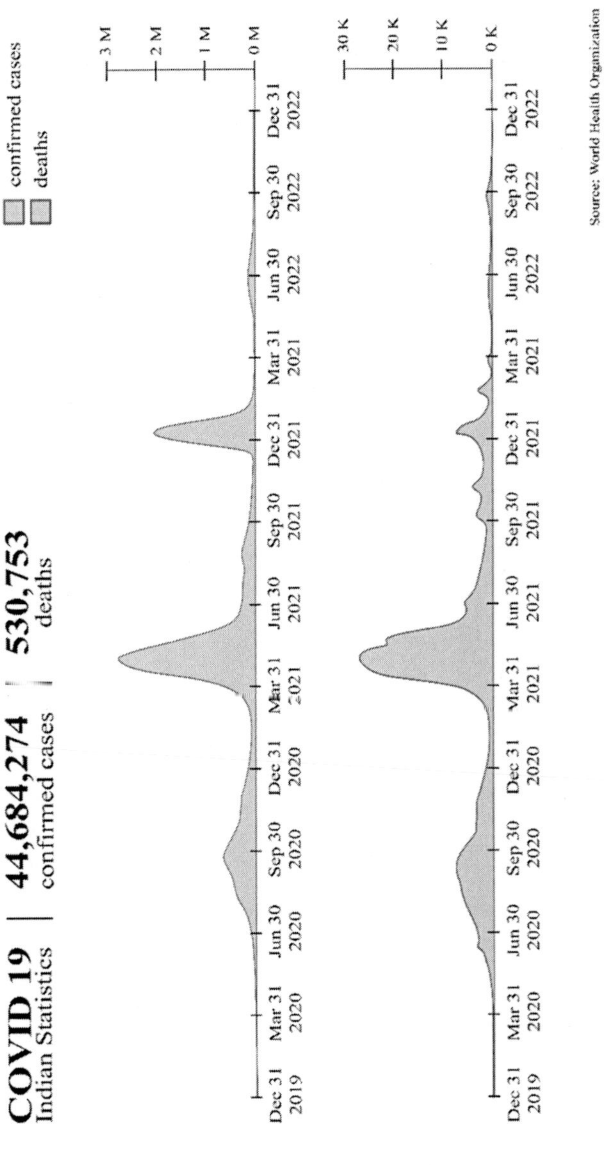

Fig 4. Indian data set for confirmed cases and death cases

At the regional level, the Western Pacific Region (-81%), the South-East Asia Region (-71%), the European Region (-63%), the Region of the Americas (-35%), the African Region (-20%), and the Eastern Mediterranean Region (-15%) all had a decline in the number of newly reported 28-day cases. Three regions saw a rise in the number of newly reported 28-day deaths: the Western Pacific Region (+173%), the Eastern Mediterranean Region (+29%), and the Region of the Americas (+13%). Three WHO regions had a decline in the number of deaths: South-East Asia (-62%), Africa (-45%), and Europe (-25%). At the national level, China (11 354 058 new cases; -85%), Japan (3 207 097 new cases; -20%), the United States of America (1 513 538 new cases; -16%), the Republic of Korea (1 032 801 new cases; -43%), and Brazil (459 986 new cases; -54%) reported the largest numbers of new 28-day cases. China (62 759 new deaths; +244%), the United States (14 625 new deaths; +31%), Japan (10 122 new deaths; +46%), the United Kingdom (3137 new deaths; -3%), and Brazil (2889 new deaths; -24%) reported the largest numbers of new 28-day deaths. Variant circulation varies by WHO region and country due to various circumstances, including previously circulating variations, vaccination coverage, and public health and socioeconomic activities. As of 6:14 p.m. CET on February 3, 2023, WHO had received reports of 6,817,478 COVID-19 deaths, including 754,018,841 confirmed cases. As of January 30, 2023, a total of 13,168,935,724 doses of vaccination had been administered.

Situation by Region, Country, Territory & Area

Name	Cases - cumulative total	Cases - newly reported in last 7 days	Deaths - cumulative total	Deaths - newly reported in last 7 days	Total vaccine doses administered per 100 population	Persons fully vaccinated with last dose of primary series per 100 population	Persons Boosted per 100 population
Global	754,018,841	1,063,802	6,817,478	6,447	168.95	64.85	30.61
+ By WHO Region							
+ By World Bank Income Group							
United States of America	100,941,827		1,097,246		199.72	68.56	34.79
China	98,587,415	195,563	111,760	353	235.52	86.82	54.7
India	44,683,122	685	530,741	2	159.79	68.97	16.49
France	38,431,258	28,254	160,670	299	234	78.95	60.85
Germany	37,810,147	77,952	166,016	47	232	76.42	62.66
Brazil	36,837,943	69,266	697,200	597	235.53	79.67	51.02
Japan	32,633,741	322,802	68,796	2,089	294.1	81.55	67.43
Republic of Korea	30,228,889	121,526	33,552	220	265.51	86.7	65.63

Fig 5. Situation by region, country, territory and area.

20. CONCLUSION

This chapter outlines how data science is being used in the research of the SARS-COV-2 pandemic. This illness places a tremendous amount of strain on the global economy as well as healthcare institutions. Data science is thought to be able to use better the limited healthcare resources available in today's age of procedures and technologies. We introduce data science and its applications in this chapter to assist in tackling COVID-19's various manifestations. Disease-related datasets that are readily accessible are used as community resources. Numerous dataset types are used to investigate distinct pandemic features at various sizes.

REFERENCES

1. He, Feng, Yu Deng, and Weina Li. "Coronavirus disease 2019: What we know?." *Journal of medical virology* 92.7 (2020): 719-725.
2. World Health Organization. "Coronavirus." (2020).
3. Perlman, Stanley. "Another decade, another coronavirus." *New England Journal of Medicine* 382.8 (2020): 760-762.
4. Singhal, Tanu. "A review of coronavirus disease-2019 (COVID-19)." *The Indian Journal of Paediatrics* 87.4 (2020): 281-286.
5. Dhama, Kuldeep, et al. "Coronavirus disease 2019–COVID-19." *Clinical microbiology reviews* 33.4 (2020): e00028-20.
6. Hasöksüz, Mustafa, Selcuk Kilic, and Fahriye Sarac. "Coronaviruses and sars-cov-2." *Turkish journal of medical sciences* 50.9 (2020): 549-556.
7. Wu, Di, et al. "The SARS-CoV-2 outbreak: what we know." *International Journal of infectious diseases* 94 (2020): 44-48.
8. Lu, Xiaoxia, et al. "SARS-CoV-2 infection in children." *New England Journal of Medicine* 382.17 (2020): 1663-1665.
9. Ludwig, Stephan, and Alexander Zarbock. "Coronaviruses and SARS-CoV-2: a brief overview." *Anaesthesia and analgesia* (2020).
10. Krammer, Florian. "SARS-CoV-2 vaccines in development." *Nature* 586.7830 (2020): 516-527.
11. Mackay, Ian M., and Katherine E. Arden. "MERS coronavirus: diagnostics, epidemiology and transmission." *Virology Journal* 12.1 (2015): 1-21.
12. Mackay, Ian M., and Katherine E. Arden. "MERS coronavirus: diagnostics, epidemiology and transmission." *Virology Journal* 12.1 (2015): 1-21.

13. Ciotti, Marco, et al. "The COVID-19 pandemic." *Critical Reviews in clinical laboratory sciences*, 57-6 (2020): 365-388.
14. Yuki, Koichi, Miho Fujiogi, and Sophia Koutsogiannaki. "COVID-19 pathophysiology: A review." *Clinical Immunology* 215 (2020): 108427.
15. Velavan, Thirumalaisamy P., and Christian G. Meyer. "The COVID-19 epidemic." *Tropical Medicine & international health* 25.3 (2020): 278.
16. Daniel, Sir John. "Education and the COVID-19 pandemic." *Prospects* 49.1 (2020): 91-96.

CHAPTER 5

A LOW-COST, PH-SENSITIVE COLOURIMETRIC PAPER-BASED DEVICE FOR THE DETECTION OF UREA

SMRITI SINHA, AKASHLINA BASU, SOUMEN DAS

Biosensors and Microfluidics Lab, School of Medical Science and Technology, IIT Kharagpur, West Bengal -721302, India

ABSTRACT

Long-term consumption of urea adulterated milk causes toxic effects on the kidney and gastrointestinal tract. Furthermore, the leakage of urea from agricultural land to water bodies leads to an imbalance in the water ecosystem. Such water intake may lead to serious health complications for humans and animals. Considering the detrimental effect of urea on human and animal health, many methods have been developed to quantify urea concentration in water or milk. This chapter intends to provide insight into conventional urea detection methods and propose a new cost-effective, simple approach that the common population can use without prior training. Conventional methods of urea testing are costly and infrastructure dependent, making them unsuitable for day-to-day utilisation for the masses. Therefore, we developed an affordable and portable paper-based colourimetric sensor to measure urea concentration in an aqueous solution. A laser printer was employed to fabricate paper devices. Experimental results showed that 8 minutes of reaction time is needed for the optimal reaction between urea and urease enzyme in the presence of a pH indicator. A strong negative correlation (r = -0.99) was obtained between the detection spot's magenta intensity and urea concentration. This device exhibits linear behaviour for the urea concentration range: 0 - 41.6 mM, with R2 = 0.98. The sensitivity of the developed device is 2.8 a.u./mM with a limit of detection of 2.92 mM. The proposed device is easy to fabricate and can be used as a disposable urea sensor, especially for initial screening purposes in resource-constrained settings.

Keywords: *urea detection, paper-based device, colourimetric sensor, pH indicator, laserjet printer*

1. INTRODUCTION

1.1 Urea and its Uses

Urea or carbamide, a compound found in mammalian urine and blood, plays a vital role in the nitrogen cycle (Higgins, 2016). Additionally, it is present in mammalian milk at levels of 7 to 20 mgdL-1. Milk is considered a wholesome food due to its intrinsic nutritional worth, and its consumption is rising annually due to a global trend toward healthy lifestyles. To meet demand and supply chain and make more profit, some milk traders engage in the unethical practice of adulteration. Urea is also an adulterant in synthetic milk production to enhance its non-protein nitrogen content (Handford, Campbell, and Elliott 2016). Besides the dairy industry, this important bio-component is also used in agriculture to gain financial gain. It is in high demand as a fertiliser in agriculture due to its high nitrogen content and ability to promote the fast growth of crops (Koundal & Kadyan, 2021).

1.2 Side Effects of Excessive Use of Urea

Regular milk consumption adulterated with urea can cause acute and chronic harmful effects on human health. It is detrimental to the human gastrointestinal tract and contributes to liver and kidney toxicity. It also results in hormone imbalance and impaired reproductive health for human consumers. Moreover, its excessive intake causes irreversible body protein modifications, contributing to a high risk of death in dialysis patients (Kumar & Dash, 2021)(Reddy, Venkatesh, and Reddy, 2017). Similarly, excessive use of urea as fertilizer affects soil pH, further reducing future crop quality. In addition, the crops produced are of subpar nutritional value, subject to pest activities.

Additionally, the accidental flow of urea from the farmland into water bodies harms the aquatic ecosystem (Maleva et al., 2013)(Sassine et al., 2021). In cattle, a dosage of urea salts from the urea-contaminated feed and water as low as 0.3 g/kg can cause toxicosis on consumption. This further results in a CNS disorder called “bovine bonkers syndrome” that makes cattle exhibit hyper-irritability, spasms, convulsions, and trembling.

This toxicity is even passed on to nursing calves through milk (Toxicosis & Poisoning, 2022). Therefore, urea detection and quantitative estimation are essential for milk and water quality control and environmental monitoring. Getting safe drinking water and food is the right of every person, so it is urgent to develop a low-cost, simple urea sensor that can be used by the common population daily to check the drinking water and milk quality.

1.3 Conventional Method for Detection and Estimation of Urea Concentration

The conventional method of urea determination mainly utilizes spectrophotometric, electrochemical, and colourimetry methods (Watt & Chrisp, 1954) (Arain et al., 2016)(Langenfeld, Payne, and Bugbee, 2021). Each method has advantages and limitations based on the material type, complexity, and final applications.

1.3.1 Spectroscopic method

A variety of spectroscopic techniques have been explored for the detection of urea. UV Visible spectroscopy-based detection (Bojic, Radovanovic, and Dimitrijevic 2008) of urea involves measuring the absorbance of the yellow-green colour complex developed when an aqueous solution of urea reacts with p-dimethylamino benzaldehyde in the presence of dilute hydrochloric acid. Additionally, a method for estimating urea concentration was developed based on the absorption peak area of the C-N and C=O bond of urea under a mid-infrared ray(Yang, Liu, and Xu 2011). Other spectroscopic methods reported for urea concentration estimation include gas chromatography-mass spectrometry (Tserng & Kalhan, 1982), Near Infrared Raman (NIR) spectroscopy (Khan et al., 2015), and fluorescence spectroscopy (Yin et al., 2021). Because of their chemical specificity, the spectroscopic-based method for urea detection provides results with an ultra-low detection limit (LoD) with good sensitivity, selectivity, and accuracy. However, most of them depend on bulky equipment, trained human resources, and planned infrastructure, making them unsuitable for use by the untrained common public.

1.3.2 Electrochemical method

The electrochemical method of urea estimation mainly involves potentiometric and amperometric sensors. It is carried out using three electrode systems: a working electrode, a reference electrode, and a counter electrode. In a potentiometric urea sensor (Trivedi et al., 2009), urea-specific urease enzymes hydrolyze urea and produce ammonia ions. Released ammonia ions create a potential difference between the working electrode and the sensor's reference electrode, which is further measured using an electrochemical analyzer. On the other hand, amperometric urea sensors (Pizzariello et al., 2001) utilize the measurement of current change between the reference electrode and working electrode due to the production of ammonium ions. Although the electrochemical method of urea sensing provides good LoD often susceptible to interference due to interfering ions present in samples and standards. Additionally, Electrochemical analyzers are expensive (~400 USD), require expertise, and are impractical for the common population to use for daily purposes for urea testing.

1.3.3 Colourimetric method

The colourimetric analytical method demonstrates the distinct colour change when analytes of interest react with their specific reagents. Based on the procedure followed, colourimetric sensing of urea is divided into Direct and Indirect methods.

1.3.3.1 Direct colourimetric method of urea sensing

The direct method of urea sensing is based on the reaction between urea and diacetyl monoxime and was first reported by Fearon WR in 1939 (Fearon, 1939). Urea reacts with diacetyl monoxime and produces a colour complex in the presence of phosphoric acid, thiosemicarbazide, sulfuric acid, and ferric chloride (Langenfeld, Payne, and Bugbee 2021). This resultant colour complex exhibit a peak absorbance at 520 nm. This approach is appropriate for determining millimolar amounts of urea in wastewater due to the absence of observable interferences. Since diacetyl monoxime must be heated continuously at the same temperature to be hydrolyzed into diacetyl, this approach necessitates the use of basic laboratory equipment; thus, this method is not appropriate for daily usage by general people.

1.3.3.2 pH-sensitive urea sensor / indirect colourimetric method of urea sensing

Indirect colourimetric methods of urea determination are based on the colour change of Phenol red (a pH indicator dye) caused by the alkalinisation of the media due to a reaction between urea and urease enzymes (Werkmeister, Koide, and Nickel 2016). A pH indicator is a compound that shows colour change upon variation in the pH of the solution. Upon interaction with Urease enzymes, urea first hydrolyses into ammonium carbamate and further hydrolyses to produce another ammonia molecule (NH_3) and carbon dioxide (CO_2). The release of NH_3, which is naturally alkaline, increases the pH of the solution.

$$CO(NH_2)_2 + H_2O\ 2NH_3 + CO_2\ (1) \quad \xrightarrow[\text{Urease enzyme}]{}$$

In the presence of phenol red dye, the resulting urea-urease complex shifts from yellow to magenta. Since the indirect method of urea sensing depends upon the pH of the resulting complex, it is called pH sensitive urea sensor. Typically UV visible spectroscopy is used to measure urea concentration based on the absorption peak and intensity of urea- urease complex in the presence of Phenol red (Bergmeyer, 2012)(Soni, Surana, and Jha, 2018). The techniques above require bulky equipment and a trained workforce. Using sophisticated UV visible spectroscopy is not feasible for the untrained common population daily. These reasons call for new inventions involving simple and affordable technology that can be made available to the masses without inconvenience. These drawbacks of traditional methods were the motivation to move towards a low-cost and low-volume alternative, paper-based devices.

1.4 Paper devices

Paper is a thin sheet of cellulose networks found abundantly in our day-to-day lives. Since the inception of papyrus, the paper has been used as a writing medium, a means of art preservation, photographing history in action, and packaging material. It has now found a purpose as a substrate for sensors in modern-day research, as the world is evolving from lab-based assays to on-the-spot detection strategies. The majority of currently available sensor technology requires expensive substrates and time-consuming fabrication processes. Paper substrates, in comparison, are very cost-efficient and demonstrate compatibility with the sensing of many organic and inorganic samples. Furthermore, the set guideline by WHO for on-the-spot analysis of analytes states that devices must follow the REASSURED criteria- real-time connectivity, ease of access, affordable, sensitive, specific, user-friendly, rapid, equipment-free, and deliverable to users (Smith et al., 2018). Paper devices fulfil all these criteria by being a low-cost alternative easily transportable to remote locations for diagnostic necessities.

1.4.1 Mechanism of fluid transport through the paper substrate

Microfluidic flow through paper substrates is influenced by different factors than traditional microfluidic channels. The most important of these factors is capillary flow in the paper, which eliminates the requirement for external pumping devices. The wicking ability of the paper determines the capillary flow rate and decays exponentially with time because the fluid evaporates as it flows through the paper. Pore volume and pore size are also important considerations when choosing a paper type for an assay. Pore size influences sample spread on paper. Pore volume defines the paper's thickness, which directly impacts the amount of sample to be added to the assay. When the spread of coloured complexes is high and deeper diffusion is present, a larger volume is required, and the colour intensity of the developed complex is less intense (Pelton, 2009).

1.4.2 Lucas-Washburn equation

The Washburn equation governs capillary flow in a paper substrate (Gardner, 1921) that deals with the interfacial surface tensions due to solid-liquid, solid-vapour, and liquid-vapour interaction of fluids while travelling through paper. θ represents the contact angle of the solid-liquid interface. The interfacial surface tension is represented by γ, and the average pore radius is given by 'r_a'. This equation predicts wetted region length, $l(t)$ of the paper after time t for a fluid with viscosity μ and tortuosity (τ) effect of capillary flow.

$$l(t) = \sqrt{\frac{r_a \gamma \cos(\theta)}{2\mu\tau^2}}\sqrt{t} \qquad (2)$$

1.4.3 Paper-based colourimetric sensor

The invention of colourimetric paper-based sensors started with paper chromatography and pH paper in the early 20th century. When the Nobel Prize in Chemistry was awarded to Martin and Synge in 1952, the research in paper sensors gained a lot of interest. The use of paper material for developing devices for performing low-cost analytical assays was first introduced in 2007 (Martinez et al., 2007a). This new development of paper sensors called μPads has since brought revolutionary perspectives to low-cost and low-volume sensor development. Paper sensors generally work on the principle of Beer-Lambert's law. When certain chemical species interact on paper, this new compound's absorbed wavelength changes. This colour intensity is then captured by the camera under controlled light conditions and analysed in image processing software like ImageJ. The analysis includes various pre-processing steps, after which the images are quantified into numerical values according to the chosen colour-space, i.e., RGB and HIS (Soda & Bakker, 2019). The advantage of using paper-based colourimetric sensors lies in their simplicity and ability to enable the user for qualitative determination of analyte concentration by analysing the colour change of detection spot through the naked eye.

1.4.4 Fabrication mechanism of the paper-based device

Due to the inherent capillary nature of paper and its hydrophilicity, it allows uncontrolled fluid flow in arbitrary directions. Fluid flow on a paper surface can be controlled by creating hydrophobic barriers using various hydrophobic materials such as resins, waxes, and polymers. These boundaries enclose a hydrophilic area, allowing reagent and analytes solution to flow along the hydrophilic spot and react with each other on the detection spot. Several methods developed for fabricating paper-based devices are discussed below.

1.4.4.1 Photolithography

The photolithography method (Martinez et al., 2007b) creates a hydrophobic boundary on paper using SU-8 photoresist. The paper was initially impregnated with SU-8 polymer by baking on a hot plate, followed by UV light treatment with an attached patterned mask. Next, the paper device was heated further on a hot plate and then washed with acetone to create a patterned device with hydrophobic and hydrophilic regions. Although this fabrication method had an exceptional resolution, the cost of the photoresist led researchers to hunt for substitutes.

1.4.4.2 Stamping method

Patterned stamps (De Tarso Garcia et al., 2014) made of rubber and metal can be used to imprint designs for hydrophobic and hydrophilic areas on the paper. Polymers, resins, and paraffin can be coated on the stamp's positive pattern and transferred onto the paper substrate forming hydrophobic areas. Due to manual handling, this method is not suitable for the mass fabrication of the paper device

1.4.4.3 Wax printing

Xerox Color Qube wax printers (Carrilho, Martinez, and Whitesides 2009) were utilised to fabricate the paper device. After heating the paper with the wax pattern, wax gets melted and spread through the paper's pores, creating hydrophilic/hydrophobic contrast on the paper substrate. This approach had a high throughput and was time-effective, although the boundaries lacked sharp edges. Xerox has now discontinued these printers. Moreover, wax boundaries are unstable against organic solvents and surfactants.

1.4.4.4 Inkjet printing

This technique fabricates the paper device using customised liquid ink and an inkjet printer. Contactless dispensing of picoliter ink in the predefined pattern is performed on a paper substrate. Upon heating for the optimized duration, it creates hydrophilic-hydrophobic contrast on the paper substrate. Although this method is quick, precise, and appropriate for the mass production of the paper device, it requires manual modification of the printer before fabrication (Abe, Suzuki, and Citterio 2008).

1.4.4.5 Laserjet printing

TLaserjet printers were first introduced in 2019 for fabricating paper-based devices to overcome the limitation of inkjet printing (Ghosh et al., 2019). Laserjet printer toner contains the hydrophobic styrene polymer that gets melted when heated above its melting temperature. Polymer permeates into paper pores on heating the patterned paper and creates stable hydrophobic regions around the hydrophilic spot. Compared to inkjet printing, this process is simple, effective, and affordable for producing large numbers of paper devices without changing the printer's factory settings.

In the present work, a paper-based colourimetric sensor has been developed for urea concentration measurement. Our research used the commonly available commercial laserjet printer for paper device fabrication. The detection mechanism is that the colour of the pH indicator changes with the increase in pH of the media, as the urease enzyme catalyses the hydrolysis of urea to shift the media pH. The change in urea concentration causes variation in the colour intensity of the detection spot. A regression-based analysis has been performed to obtain an equation relating to urea concentration and colour intensity. The colour change of the detection spot can be observed visually, and actual urea concentration can be estimated using the developed equation. Further, the sensitivity, detection limits, and quantification limits were calculated. This device is simple, affordable, easy to fabricate, and requires a small sample volume. This paper-based sensor offers the possibility to evaluate urea concentration for diagnosis, environmental monitoring, and quality control purpose in resource-limited settings.

2. FABRICATION AND PREPARATION OF A PAPER-BASED DEVICE FOR UREA ESTIMATION

Device patterns were designed using open-source Inkscape tools. The pattern was printed on cellulose paper, Whatman filter paper Grade #1 [pore size: 11μm] by using a Laserjet printer (Hp 1020 plus). Overall, device fabrication and preparation are summarily illustrated in Fig.1. The *fabrication technique* employs the toner particles of the laser printer as hydrophobic material for fabricating the hydrophobic barriers surrounding the desired hydrophilic detection spot on the paper substrate. In contrast to wax printing, this method is simpler and more economical for mass-scale paper device fabrication. Subsequently, the pattern-printed paper is heated at 165 °C for 20 minutes. Printed polymer melts and wicks laterally and vertically on the porous paper during heating, thus generating a well-defined hydrophilic area surrounded by a hydrophobic boundary across the paper thickness.

Following the procedure mentioned above, the fabricated paper device was further prepared for detecting urea in an aqueous solution. A reagent solution specific to urea detection was prepared by mixing 13.5 mg urease, 200 μl of Phenol Red, and 200 μl of Phosphate buffer (pH 6.8). The detection spot of the device was functionalised with 5μl of reagent solution. After drying for 10-15 minutes, a 5 μl of aqueous urea solution was spotted in the detection spot. Colour change at the detection spot was captured using a digital camera (Nikon, Japan) under controlled lighting conditions. Image analysis was performed using Matlab® tools.

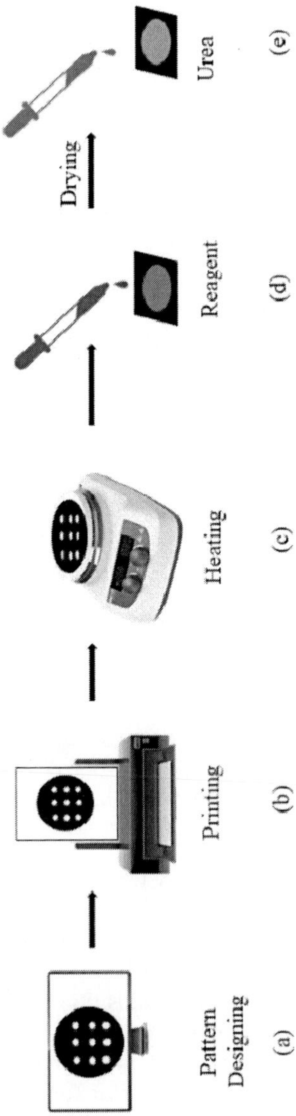

Figure 1. Schematic demonstrating the procedure of preparing paper sensors. (a) Designing the paper sensor on Inkscape tools, (b) printing the design on paper using a laser toner printer, (c) heating the paper device at an optimised temperature to allow the formation of hydrophobic boundaries, (d) adding a reagent of choice to the detection spot, (e) adding the analyte to the detection spot for colour development

3. RESULTS AND DISCUSSION

3.1 reaction time optimization

The development of the magenta colour on the detection spot is linked with an enzymatic process, which requires an optimal time to develop colour. There is a gradual change in colour over time, depending on its reaction process. Therefore, optimisation of the reaction time is necessary. A 5 µl of reagent solution containing urease enzyme and Phenol red was added to the detection spot and dried at room temperature. After drying, a 5µl of 41.6 millimolar (mM) urea solution was added to the detection spot. Colour change at the detection spot was captured for 0-20 minutes.

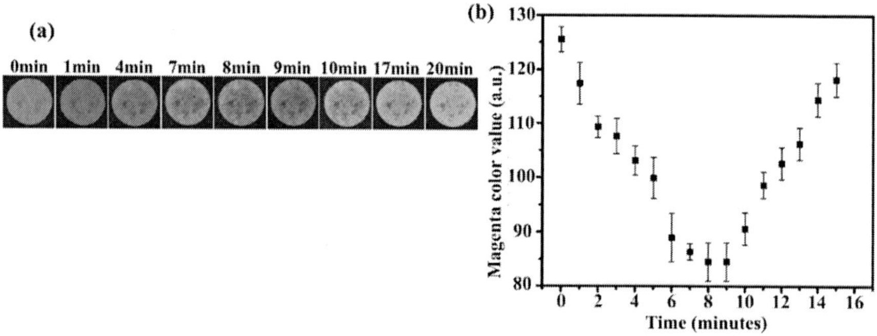

Figure 2. (a) Colour change over time on the reaction between 41.6 mM urea solution and urease-phenol red mixture; (b) Variation of the Magenta colour value of the detection spot versus reaction time. The error bar represents the standard deviation (s.d.) of five measurements.

The optimal reaction time was determined by measuring the Magenta colour value of the captured image. As shown in Fig 2(a), with the reaction time of 0~ 8 min, the magenta colour develops and becomes deeper but remains approximately constant until 9 minutes. Beyond 9 min, the detection spot begins to show a transition toward yellow colour. This indicates a minimum of 8 minutes of reaction time is required for optimum colour development on the paper device, and catalytic activity of the urease enzyme declines after 9 min of reaction. In Fig. 2(b), the Magenta colour value of the detection spot for the time was presented. It could be observed from the plot that the magenta colour value decreases till 8 min of reaction due to the development of deeper magenta colour with time and then tends to saturate on 9 minutes. However, when the reaction time exceeds 9 min, the intensity increases due to turning the detection spot yellow. Therefore, in the subsequent study, the image was captured after 8 minutes of adding urea to the detection spot.

3.2 Analytical Performance

After determining the optimal reaction time, the analytical performance of the developed device for urea measurement was examined. A reagent solution containing urease enzyme and phenol red was spotted in the detection spot. After drying for 10 minutes, a standard aqueous urea solution with a concentration ranging from 0 -167 mM was spotted in the detection spot. The image was captured for 8 minutes, and the magenta colour value was analysed (Fig 3 (a)). The increase in urea concentration possibly causes more urea hydrolysis, thus producing more ammonia and significantly increasing solution pH. Consequently, the colour indicator, Phenol red, shows a progression towards magenta from yellow as the alkalinity of media increases with an increase in urea concentration.

Fig. 3(b) shows the magenta value of the detection spot with urea concentration ranging from 0 to 167 Mm. Magenta colour becomes darker and, consequently, its value decreases with increasing urea concentration and tends to saturate beyond 125mM of urea. Evaluation of the correlation between magenta colour and urea concentration reveals a strong negative correlation with Pearson's coefficient, $r = -0.99$. It is found that magenta colour value and urea in the concentration range of 0 – 41.6 mM are linearly related as $Y = -2.8X + 207.7$, with $R^2 = 0.98$, as shown in Fig. 3(c) using the regression method. (Note that each data point represents average magenta colour values obtained from five repeated experiment sets). The slope of the proposed equation indicates that the magenta colour value decreased by 2.8 units per millimolar change in urea concentration. The limits of detection (LoD) calculated using 3.3sd/*S* criteria, where *S* is the slope, and sd is the standard deviation of the y-intercept of the regression line, n=5 was 2.92mM. The quantification limit (10sd/*S*) was 8.86mM. This device's linear response and detection limit are good enough to make it suitable for detecting urea contamination in drinking water. In the future, the sensitivity of this device can be enhanced to detect the ultra-low level of urea contamination in real samples.

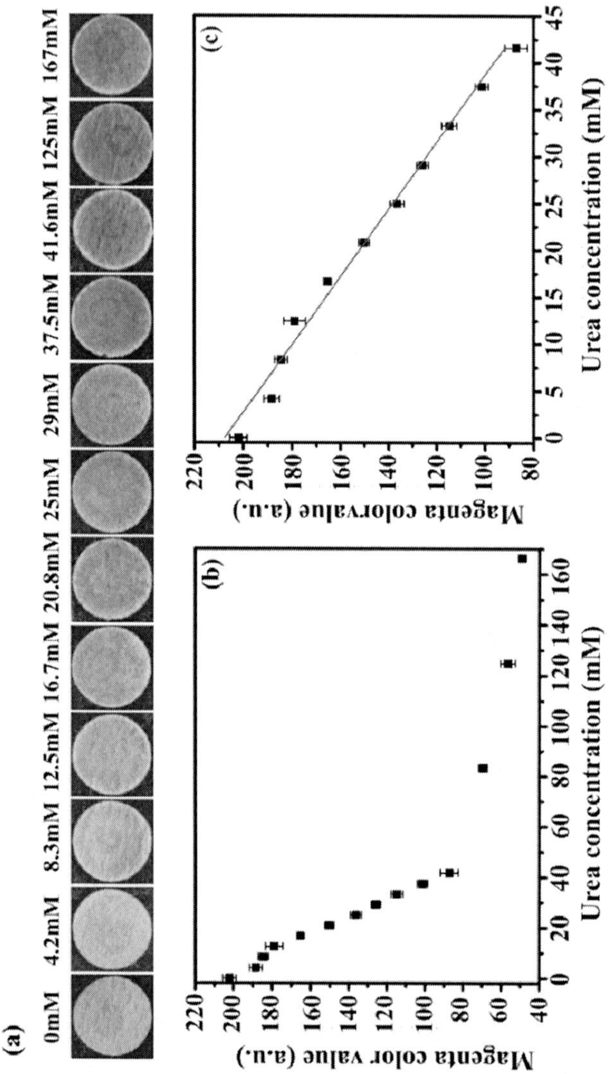

Figure 3. (a) Variation of colour and intensity of paper device detection spot with different urea concentration; (b) The detecting spot magenta value for urea concentration, which ranges from 0 to 167 mM; (c) Linear regression fit line of the data ($R^2 = 0.98$) with urea concentration ranging from 0 to 42 mM. The error bar represents the standard deviation of the result from five sets of repeated experiments.

3.3 Disposability of Developed Paper Device

Incineration allows the developed paper device to be conveniently disposed of after use. This can be done within a minute, which produces little residue, making it an environment-friendly approach.

4. CONCLUSIONS

In summary, a simple and rapid paper-based device for estimating urea concentration in artificial samples with a pH-sensitive colourimetric procedure was successfully developed. Laserjet printing was employed for creating the hydrophilic-hydrophobic pattern on paper with minimal cost and high throughput. This device is based on the principle that the colour and intensity of the urea-urease reaction derivative will change significantly with the change in pH of the solution. Experimental analysis revealed that the urea-urease reaction is a time-dependent process. A correlation and regression analysis has been performed to develop an equation relating the resulting magenta colour value and urea concentration. The detection spot's magenta colour was negatively correlated (r= -0.99) with urea concentration. This device can successfully estimate the urea concentration in the range of 0-41.6 mM and obtained LoD of 2.92 mM is good enough for the initial urea screening of a sample in resource-limited settings. The proposed device might be helpful for a layperson to visually examine urea concentration in water or milk daily. On further validation with the real samples, the proposed device potentially aids in environmental monitoring, diagnostic purpose, and food quality control.

ACKNOWLEDGMENTS

I acknowledge the Biosensors and Microfluidics Lab, SMST, IIT Kharagpur, for providing the fabrication and characterisation facilities.

REFERENCES

1. Abe, Koji, Koji Suzuki, and Daniel Citterio. 2008. "Inkjet-Printed Microfluidic Multianalyte Chemical Sensing Paper." *Analytical Chemistry* 80 (18): 6928–34. https://doi.org/10.1021/ac800604v.
2. Arain, M., Ayman Nafady, Z. H. I., Syed Tufail Hussain Sherazi, T. S., Hamayun Khan, A. A., Abdul Niaz, & Magnus Willander. (2016). "Simpler and Highly Sensitive Enzyme-Free Sensing of Urea via NiO Nanostructures Modified Electrode." *RSC Advances* 6 (45): 39001–6.

3. Bergmeyer, Hans-Ulrich. 2012. *Methods of Enzymatic Analysis*. Elsevier.
4. Bojic, Jorgovanka, Blaga Radovanovic, and Jasmina Dimitrijevic. 2008. "Spectrophotometric Determination of Urea in Dermatologic Formulations and Cosmetics." *Analytical Sciences* 24 (6): 769–74.
5. Carrilho, Emanuel, Andres W. Martinez, and George M. Whitesides. 2009. "Understanding Wax Printing: A Simple Micropatterning Process for Paper-Based Microfluidics." *Analytical Chemistry* 81 (16): 7091–95. https://doi.org/10.1021/ac901071p.
6. Fearon, William Robert. 1939. "The Carbamido Diacetyl Reaction: A Test for Citrulline." *Biochemical Journal* 33 (6): 902.
7. Gardner, W. (1921). "Note on the Dynamics of Capillary Flow." *Physical Review* 18 (3): 206–9. https://doi.org/10.1103/PhysRev.18.206.
8. Ghosh, Rajesh, Saranya Gopalakrishnan, Rangasamy Savitha, Thiruvengadam Renganathan, and Subramanium Pushpavanam. 2019. "Fabrication of Laser Printed Microfluidic Paper-Based Analytical Devices (LP-MPADs) for Point-of-Care Applications." *Scientific Reports* 9 (1): 1–11. https://doi.org/10.1038/s41598-019-44455-1.
9. Handford, C. E, Katrina Campbell, & Christopher T Elliott. (2016). "Impacts of Milk Fraud on Food Safety and Nutrition with Special Emphasis on Developing Countries." *Comprehensive Reviews in Food Science and Food Safety* 15 (1): 130–42.
10. Higgins, C. (2016). "Urea and the Clinical Value of Measuring Blood Urea Concentration." *Acutecaretesting. Org*, pp. 1–6.
11. Khan, Khan Mohammad, Hemant Krishna, Shovan Kumar Majumder, & Pradeep Kumar Gupta. (2015). "Detection of Urea Adulteration in Milk Using Near-Infrared Raman Spectroscopy." *Food Analytical Methods* 8: pp. 93–102.
12. Koundal, Deepika, and Virendar Kadyan. 2021. "Urea Spreaders for Improving the Crop Productivity in Agriculture: Recent Developments." *Smart Agriculture Automation Using Advanced Technologies*, 195–206.
13. Kumar, V., & Susmita Dash. (2021). "Evaporation-Based Low-Cost Method for the Detection of Adulterant in Milk." *ACS Omega* 6 (41): 27200–207.
14. Langenfeld, Noah James, Lauren Elizabeth Payne, and Bruce Bugbee. 2021. "Colorimetric Determination of Urea Using Diacetyl Monoxime with Strong Acids." *Plos One* 16 (11): e0259760.

15. Maleva, Maria, Galina Borisova, Nadezda Chukina, Galina Nekrasova, and M N V Prasad. 2013. "Influence of Exogenous Urea on Photosynthetic Pigments, 14CO2 Uptake, and Urease Activity in Elodea Densa—Environmental Implications." *Environmental Science and Pollution Research* 20 (9): 6172–77.
16. Martinez, Andres W, Scott T Phillips, Manish J Butte, George M Whitesides, W Martinez, S T Phillips, M J Butte, and G M Whitesides. 2007a. "Patterned Paper as a Platform for Inexpensive, Low-Volume, Portable Bioassays**." *Angew. Chem. Int. Ed* 46: 1318–20. https://doi.org/10.1002/anie.200603817.
17. Pelton, R. (2009). "Bioactive Paper Provides a Low-Cost Platform for Diagnostics." *TrAC - Trends in Analytical Chemistry* 28 (8): 925–42. https://doi.org/10.1016/j.trac.2009.05.005.
18. Pizzariello, Andrea, Miroslav Stredanský, Silvia Stredanská, and Stainslav Miertuš. 2001. "Urea Biosensor Based on Amperometric PH-Sensing with Hematein as a PH-Sensitive Redox Mediator." *Talanta* 54 (4): 763–72.
19. Reddy, D Maheswara, K Venkatesh, and C Venkata Sesha Reddy. 2017. "Adulteration of Milk and Its Detection: A Review." *International Journal of Chemical Studies* 5 (4): 613–17.
20. Sassine, Youssef N, Layla Naim, Zeina El Sebaaly, Sami Abou Fayssal, Mohammed A Alsanad, and Milena H Yordanova. 2021. "Nano Urea Effects on Pleurotus Ostreatus Nutritional Value Depending on the Dose and Timing of Application." *Scientific Reports* 11 (1): 1–11.
21. Smith, Suzanne, Jan G Korvink, Dario Mager, and Kevin Land. 2018. "The Potential of Paper-Based Diagnostics to Meet the ASSURED Criteria," 34012–34. https://doi.org/10.1039/c8ra06132g.
22. Soda, Yoshiki, and Eric Bakker. 2019. "Quantification of Colorimetric Data for Paper-Based Analytical Devices." *ACS Sensors* 4 (12): 3093–3101.
23. Soni, A., Rajat Kumar Surana, & Sandeep Kumar Jha. (2018). "Smartphone-Based Optical Biosensor for the Detection of Urea in Saliva." *Sensors and Actuators B: Chemical* 269: pp. 346–53.
24. Tarso Garcia, Paulo De, Thiago Miguel Garcia Cardoso, Carlos Diego Garcia, Emanuel Carrilho, and Wendell Karlos Tomazelli Coltro. 2014. "A Handheld Stamping Process to Fabricate Microfluidic Paper-Based Analytical Devices with Chemically Modified Surface for Clinical Assays." *RSC Advances* 4 (71): 37637–44. https://doi.org/10.1039/c4ra07112c.

25. Toxicosis, Ammonia, and Urea Poisoning. 2022. "Non-protein Nitrogen Poisoning in Animals," 2–6.
26. Trivedi, U B, D Lakshminarayana, I L Kothari, N G Patel, H N Kapse, K K Makhija, P B Patel, and C J Panchal. 2009. "Potentiometric Biosensor for Urea Determination in Milk." *Sensors and Actuators B: Chemical* 140 (1): 260–66.
27. Tserng, Kou Yi, and Satish C Kalhan. 1982. "Gas Chromatography/Mass Spectrometric Determination of [15N] Urea in Plasma and Application to Urea Metabolism Study." *Analytical Chemistry* 54 (3): 489–91.
28. Watt, G. W, & Joseph D Chrisp. (1954). "Spectrophotometric Method for Determination of Urea." *Analytical Chemistry* 26 (3): 452–53.
29. Werkmeister, F X, T Koide, and B A Nickel. 2016. "Ammonia Sensing for Enzymatic Urea Detection Using Organic Field Effect Transistors and a Semipermeable Membrane." *Journal of Materials Chemistry B* 4 (1): 162–68.
30. Yang, Ren-Jie, Rong Liu, and Ke-Xin Xu. 2011. "Adulteration Detection of Urea in Milk by Mid-Infrared Spectroscopy." *Spectroscopy and Spectral Analysis* 31 (9): 2383–85.
31. Yin, Wenzhi, Ye Zhang, Jiao Gu, Tingyu Wang, Chaoqun Ma, Chun Zhu, Lei Li, Zichen Yang, Tuo Zhu, and Guoqing Chen. 2021. "Urea Detection in Milk by Urease-Assisted PH-Sensitive Carbon Dots." *Applied Optics* 60 (33): 10421–28.

CHAPTER 6

DEVELOPMENT OF SENSOR-BASED HYBRID TYPE MINE WATER TREATMENT METHODOLOGY TO REDUCE THE EFFECTS OF HEXAVALENT CHROMIUM: A CONCEPTUAL STUDY

MANISHA DAS, FALGUNI SARKAR

Department of Mining Engineering, National Institute of Technology, Rourkela, India, Pin: 769008

ABSTRACT

The release of heavy metals from mining areas more than the allowable limit causes severe environmental pollution by contaminating nearby water sources and soil. In this context, Chromium released from chromite mines generally causes a major health hazard from the perspective of carcinogenic, genotoxic, and non-biodegradable characteristics. Undesirable health effects allied with Cr-VI exposure include work-related asthma, eye irritation, perforated eardrums, respiratory disorders, kidney problems, liver damage, pulmonary congestion, skin irritation, corrosion and staining of the teeth etc. Furthermore, hexavalent chromium [Cr-VI] is more toxic if inhaled or can enter the human body from drinking water sources. Hence, it is imperative to build apposite treatment strategies for the hexavalent Chromium, considering the regulatory threshold limit (0.05mg/l). In this context, numerous procedures, viz. solvent-extraction, adsorption using activated carbon, clay, biomass, electrochemical reduction, and bioremediation, have been successfully experimented with worldwide. But the major problems encountered during the selection of appropriate technology in respect of economic feasibility, the system's efficacy, the volume of water to be handled and the quality of water. This paper discusses the chemical features and toxicity of Cr-VI, and all the possible methods implemented effectively for eliminating Cr-VI from contaminated water in mining areas have been studied. Accordingly, a sensor-based hybrid type water treatment procedure is proposed by integrating a suitable combination of adsorption and biological processes, which is expected to mitigate the harmful effects of the Cr-VI contamination.

Keywords: *Hexavalent Chromium; Carcinogenic; Adsorption; Bioremediation; solvent extraction.*

1. INTRODUCTION

The evidence of Chromium (Cr) is generally found in different water bodies due to natural and anthropogenic sources. Cr-VI is formed when Mafic and Ultramafic rocks are oxidized due to microbial action. The discharge from the metal and chemical industries is the major contributor to Cr-VI and Cr-III (i.e., hexavalent and trivalent Chromium) pollution. The oxidation states of the Chromium present could vary between -2 and +6. The Hexavalent and trivalent Chromium, which are interconvertible, are the most stable forms of Cr in water. Hence, Chromium can be found as Cr-III or Cr-VI [1]. Molecularly, the redox couple Cr-III or Cr-VI has a high E^o (Redox potential) value. In this context, Fe (II), phosphate, sulfide, and organic reagents like humic acid may be introduced to reduce Cr-VI to Cr-III for reverse transformation if required [2, 3].

The basic harmful and poisonous nature of hexavalent Cr-VI compounds can impose adverse effects on the health condition of humans as well as on other living organisms [4]. Prolonged and ongoing exposure to Cr-VI can harm the skin, eyes, blood, respiratory, and immune system, even at lower concentrations [5, 6]. There are also substantial chances of DNA damage and tumour enlargement etc., due to the genotoxic effect of Chromium [7, 8]. The increase of concentrations of Cr-VI in surrounding surface aquatic bodies and topsoil, whether due to natural or anthropogenic activities, is a serious environmental concern worldwide [9, 10, 11]. Contaminated water released by mines, steel plants, paint factories, wood and paper industries, etc., increases chromium content in adjacent water bodies [12, 13]. The incineration of coal and municipal waste also contributes to the increase in the concentration of Cr-VI in surrounding soil and surface water bodies [14].

Early research depicted that the specific chemical reduction processes, different adsorption methods and electro-coagulation are useful techniques for the elimination of Cr-VI from water. However, these methods are normally capable of eliminating higher concentrations of Cr-VI but have disadvantages like excess sludge production and the use of large amounts of harmful chemicals etc. Due to the widespread presence of microbes, bioremediation can be recognised as a viable alternative to these processes, particularly for wastewater containing a low and moderate concentration of Cr-VI [15, 16, 17].

2. CHROMIUM AND ITS SOURCES

Chromium exists in the environment with several valance states -2, -1, 0, +1, +2, +3, +4, +5, and +6. Hexavalent Cr-VI and Trivalent Cr-III are observed as the most stable state of Cr in the environment [10]. The most familiar forms of Cr-VI in water bodies are CrO_4, CrO_7, H_2CrO_4, and $HCrO_4$ etc., and the common form of Cr-III are $Cr(OH)_2+$, CrO_2+, $HCrO_2$ etc. [18]. The Chromite ore ($FeCr_2O_4$) can be recognised as the prime source of Cr-III in the surroundings. Generally, Chromite is chemically static and cannot readily dissolve in water. But microbial actions cause the Cr-III to liberate in nature from Chromite which is readily converted to Cr-VI due to oxidation. Cr-III dominates nature due to its kinetic energy and other environmental factors like pH. Still, concentrations of Cr-VI beyond permissible limits in water bodies have been recurrently tested for countering artificial pollution scenarios. Artificial use and civic sources are nearly related to the presence of Cr-VI in sediments and waters. Open dumps constructed by the solid rejects of Chromite ore processing plants frequently contaminate water resources by adding pollutants. Also, sewage and tannery sludge generally bear higher content of hexavalent Chromium, which can pollute the neighbouring water bodies. The uncontrolled and extensive use of the chromium-based product in the agrarian field is also a major source of chromium pollution. Particularly hexavalent Chromium is richly found in ashes produced by the combustion of coal, lignite, and other external solid coal-based wastes. Langard (1990) [41] observed that a large quantity of Cr-VI compound, namely Na2CrO4, was produced during the industrial processing of ferrous Chromite through lime treatment of chromite ores. This resulted in the increase of Cr-VI-based water-soluble compounds like $(CrOCl_4)^-$, *H2Cr2O7*, CrF_6, CrO_3, $Cr_2O_7^{-2}$, and H_2CrO_4 in adjacent water bodies.

3. TOXICITY

Among the major forms of Chromium, trivalent Chromium metabolises the water's lipids, glucose, and Amino acids. Whereas hexavalent chromium Cr-VI is extremely toxic even at minute concentrations. Cr-VI largely induces mutation and chromosomal breaks by binding with DNA and causes major damage to the body [19]. Exposure to Cr-VI can affect the function of the cell and can also be a reason for cancer in the lungs, kidneys, and liver in the human body. Direct contact with Cr-VI can also cause dermatitis and dermal necrosis [20]. In mining areas, carcinomas in the bronchial system can affect people, particularly labourers, exposed to Cr-VI [21]. Furthermore, cr-VI, by reducing neuronal cells causes neurotoxicity [22].

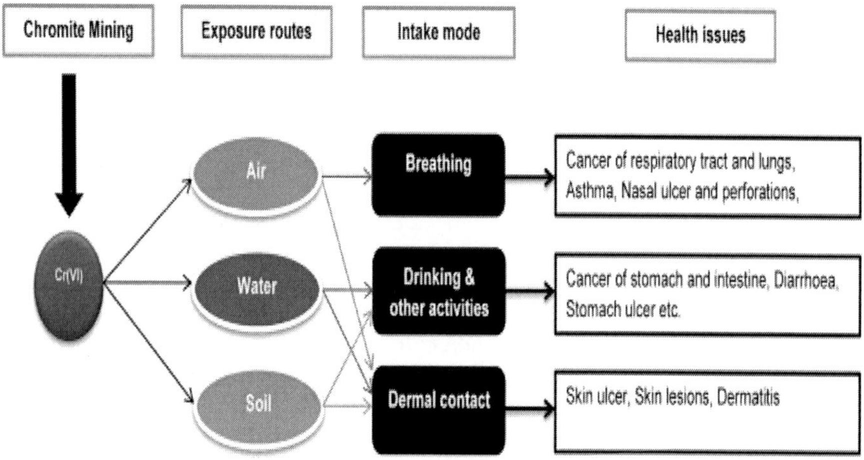

Fig 1. Sources of hexavalent Chromium [29,30]

4. SCENARIO OF THE MINE AREA UNDER CASE STUDY

A renowned chromite mine and its neighbouring area situated at Sukinda Valley in Odisha has been taken as a case study zone. The Sukinda Valley area comprises almost 97% of the chromite ore reserves of India, which plays an essential role in stainless steel, leather, and alloy production. The area is bounded by the Iron ore belt in the north, and the quartzite belt in the south, extending in the east-west direction. Chromite is the predominant ore mineral in the belt. The drainage system of the mine area is controlled by a Nalas, which is perennial. The Nalas is also fed by the water discharged from various mines. Damsala Nala is a major water source which crosses the mining area along the length. A *Nala* is one of the important sources of water for the majority of habitants for consumption of drinking. Open defecation, direct water discharge from mines during the rainy season and dumping of waste near the water source generally contaminate the water body of Nala and ground and other surface water resources. The Cr-VI concentration in the drinking water sources in the mining area is more than the permissible limit for Cr-VI, i.e. 0.05mg/l (as per BIS). According to various surveys conducted by different agencies, a large number of wells and watercourses in the case study mine area are found to be contaminated by hexavalent Chromium and containing higher Cr-VI content in 'surface water' and 'ground water' against a permissible limit of 0.05mg/l [24]. A substantial percentage of people residing in 06 nearby gram panchayats were suspected of suffering from cancer-like diseases in a cancer detection camp organized by IMFA Ltd.[42].Various studies also depicted that the residents living adjacent to the mines have no option but to drink toxic water and inhale chrome dust. Regular suffering of people from skin diseases, gas enteritis etc. may be due to the Cr-VI contamination.

5. STUDY ON RENOWNED TREATMENT PROCESSES

5.1. Reduction procedures using different chemicals: Numerous reducing agents like ferrous composites and zero-valent iron were applied in acidic media for the Cr-VI treatment of surface wastewater and ground water [2]. The most relevant procedure of Cr-VI elimination is its reduction to trivalent chromium Cr-III, leaving Cr-III hydroxide in the form of a precipitate. Besides this, the Cr-VI can be reduced by sulfur compounds viz., sulfur dioxide (SO2) and sodium bisulfite (NaHSO3) etc. [18]. Iron in its divalent/trivalent forms can also act as a reducing agent for Cr-VI reduction at low PH [25-26]. The study by Katsoyannis et al. (2020) represented an autocatalytic nature of Cr-VI during its reaction with ferrous iron. The use of well-known reducing agents like sulfur composites, hydrogen peroxide, hydrazine, sodium hydrosulfite (dithionite) etc., has shown to be less effective when used in alkaline conditions [2]. Generating a vast amount of sludge is the elementary problem of these techniques. These techniques generally need help with difficult sludge disposal problems, which incur higher financial investments and expenditures. Sludge disposals also have negative environmental attributes. Thus, there is a need to develop a novel technology to deal with these issues.

5.2. Ion Exchange is a process to treat wastewater containing heavy metals in which non-toxic ions replace the undesired ions (Shown in Fig. 2). To elevate the efficacy of removing Cr-VI from the water, various ion exchange integration methods have been implemented during the treatment procedure. During the exchange reaction, ion exchange agents showed high effectiveness via substituting Cu (II) cation from the central metal ion position [27]. Yea et al. (2019) showed Pyridine resin based on silica can remove 99.3% of hexavalent Chromium through Ion Exchange [28]. One of the proficient strategies for Cr-VI separation is the strong base anion exchange (SBA), which utilises "an inert polymeric resin actuated with face and interstitial interchangeable functional groups" [27].

5.3. Membrane filtration and Nanofiltration: Membrane filtration is an advanced technology to treat and manage heavy metals in contaminated wastewater. Due to its semi-permeability and high adaptability, it eliminates hexavalent Chromium in wastewater. Ultrafiltration, nanofiltration, and reverse osmosis are well-known membrane filtration approaches used in water treatment. Figure 2 illustrates the fundamental design of the membrane filtration technique in treating wastewater containing heavy metals. As heavy metals easily penetrate the membrane, it is not effectively used to purify water containing dissolved metal [29]. Still, an adsorptive filtration membrane can achieve the same, as it delivers a dual-function mechanism [30]. For example, an ultra-filtration membrane composed of cellulose acetate polymer, polymethyl additive and 'amine modified TiO_2' was successfully used to remove Cr-VI with a 99.8% rate [27].

5.4. Nanofiltration is an advanced membrane filtration technique used to separate various types of salt and heavy metals. An electrostatic charge on nanofiltration membrane surfaces is induced to improve ion selection. Based on a study of AFC80 on NF membrane showed a reduction in the concentration below WHO standard for safe drinking water [31]. Basaran 2015 [32] investigated 97.6% rejection of Cr-VI by NF90 membrane and 95% by NF270 membrane, respectively. Gaikwad (2017) also found that NF300 and PN40 membranes have elevated 'rejection competence' for Cr-VI removal by 97% and 88%, respectively [33]. A membrane with high rejection to seawater "(SWHR-membrane) and high rejection to brackish water (AG-membrane)" showed 91% elimination.

5.6. Adsorption. Molecular attachment to solid surfaces through physical forces/chemical bonds is called adsorption. A good adsorbent should have inbuilt characteristics like 'Mechanical strength', ample physical and chemical stability and 'exchange capacity'. The parameters influencing the adsorption rate are pH of the medium, adsorbent lozenge, contact duration and normal tendency of adulterant. Multiple investigations have been conducted to determine which reagents are better at removing organic and inorganic contaminants from water. The efficacies of the materials such as "activated carbon, agro wastes, biochar, agro-waste ash, low-cost agriculture originated material, zeolite, nanotubes, nanoparticles" etc. have been established by various researchers in this regard [27].

5.7. Biochar: Pyrolysis of high lignin-containing woody organic matter at low temperatures (200-400°C) generally produces useful biochars. The high surface charge and surface area of biochar make it highly effective for adsorbing Cr-VI (Table 1). Nowadays, the use of different types of agricultural residues, municipal wastes, industrial wastes, etc., is very common for generating biochar on an industrial scale. A scientific study has also demonstrated two-step pyrolysis for preparing biochar from corn straw and using the product to remove Cr-VI. Activating biochar resulted in higher adsorption capacity after being activated.[27].

5.8. Activated carbon is a material with high carbon content prepared physic-chemically by pretreatment of feedstock and post-treatment of biochar. Hydrothermal carbonisation, as well as pyrolysis, is observed as a useful technique for preparing carbon-rich materials. Products acquired from the hydrothermal procedure are identified as hydro char [34]. Coal, coconut shell, lignite, and wood are the frequently used feedstocks for the production of activated carbon for wastewater management.

5.9. Biological remediation or bioremediation is a process that uses living organisms like bacteria, yeast, and algae to remove contaminants and pollutants in the environment. Living organisms have been shown to act as agents capable of bioremediation. Phenomenon such as biosorption has also been used to create adsorbents from bio-originated products and by-products. Because of the involvement of bio-origination, it is termed biosorption. In this process, In the biosorption process, the elimination of impurities is influenced by the functional groups adhered to the surface of the functional bio adsorbent. Hence bacteria can ease the disposal of essence species from submarine results according to adsorptive parcels of their cellular face. The biosorption of heavy metal ions by microorganisms is affected by different aspects carrying explicit face parcels of the microorganism (biosorbent), the volume of bio-mass, physicochemical aspects of the result analogous as temperature, pH, original essence ion attention, and the actuality of other ions.

5.10. Combination of Biological processes in other existing processes

5.10.1. Biochemical: The method of using microbes and chemicals in pollutant removal is known as the biochemical process. For example, the influence of acidithiobacillus ferrooxidans and pyrites in reducing Cr-VI was investigated in research [27].

Table 1: Various Adsorbent used in Cr-VI Removal [27]

Adsorbent	Chromium (VI)	Concentration (mg/l), dose (g/l), pH, temperature (C), time (min) and shaking rate(rpm)	Adsorption capacity	Mechanism	Fitted Kinetic model	Isotherm model	References
Biochar							
distillers grains (DG)-biochar	Cr-VI	50, 1.25, 2.0, 25, 1440 and 300	8.1 mg/L	Adsorption	Pseudo-second order	Langmuir	*Lian et al. (2019)*
Phosphogypsum modified (PM)-biochar	Cr-VI	50, 1.25, 2.0, 25, 1440 and 300	38.2 mg/L	Adsorption	Pseudo-second order	Freundlich model	*Lian et al. (2019)*
Wheat straw biochar	Cr-VI	100, 1.25, 5.6, room temperature, 1440 and 160	2.4 mg/L	Adsorption			*Zhang et al. (2019)*
Wheat straw biochar-Nzvi	Cr-VI	100, 1.25, 5.6, room temperature, 1440 and 160	8.06 mg/L	Adsorption			*Zhang et al. (2019)*
Sweet lime peels biochar	Cr-VI	20, 0.50, 2.0, 30, 720 and 120	9.92 mg/L	OeH, C]O, COOH participated in Cr-VI adsorption	pseudo second order	Langmuir	*Shakya et al. (2019)*
Activated carbon							
ZnO-tetrapods/activated carbon (ZAC) nanocomposite	Cr-VI	10, 2, 2, room temperature, 420, 240	96%	Electrostatic attraction	Pseudo-second-order and Elovich model		*Sharma et al. (2019)*
ZnO-nanoparticles loaded parthenium weed activated carbon (ZnONPs-PWAC)	Cr-VI	50, 1.0, 3, -, 90, -	99%	Electrostatic interaction and chemical reaction			*Kamaraj et al. (2020)*
Polysulfide rubber (PSR) coated granular activated carbon	Cr-VI	10, 11.0, 4.0, 22, 2880, 40	100%	diffusion, electrostatic attraction by protonated polysulfide	Pseudo-second order	Langmuir model	*Mortazavian et al. (2019)*
Nano-adsorbent							
Magnetic magnetite (Fe3O4) Nanoparticles	Cr-VI	25, 1.0, 2.0, 25 and 1440,	9.69 mg/L	electrostatic attraction	pseudo-second-order	Sips and Langmuir	*Rajput et al. (2016)*

5.10.2. Constructed wetland is an advanced technology used for the management of wastewater treatment by incorporating microbes, plants, and adsorbents together, which depends on the experimental setup. There are various things which help remove the Cr-VI. Among which plants, microbes and bedding substrates are the most naturally existing ways. The plants remove the majority (i.e. 33-48%) of the Cr-VI [35]. In another investigation, the researchers deliberated that the constructed wetland planted with Leersia hexandra Swartz in association with Rhizosphere reduces 100% of Cr-VI under optimal conditions.[36].

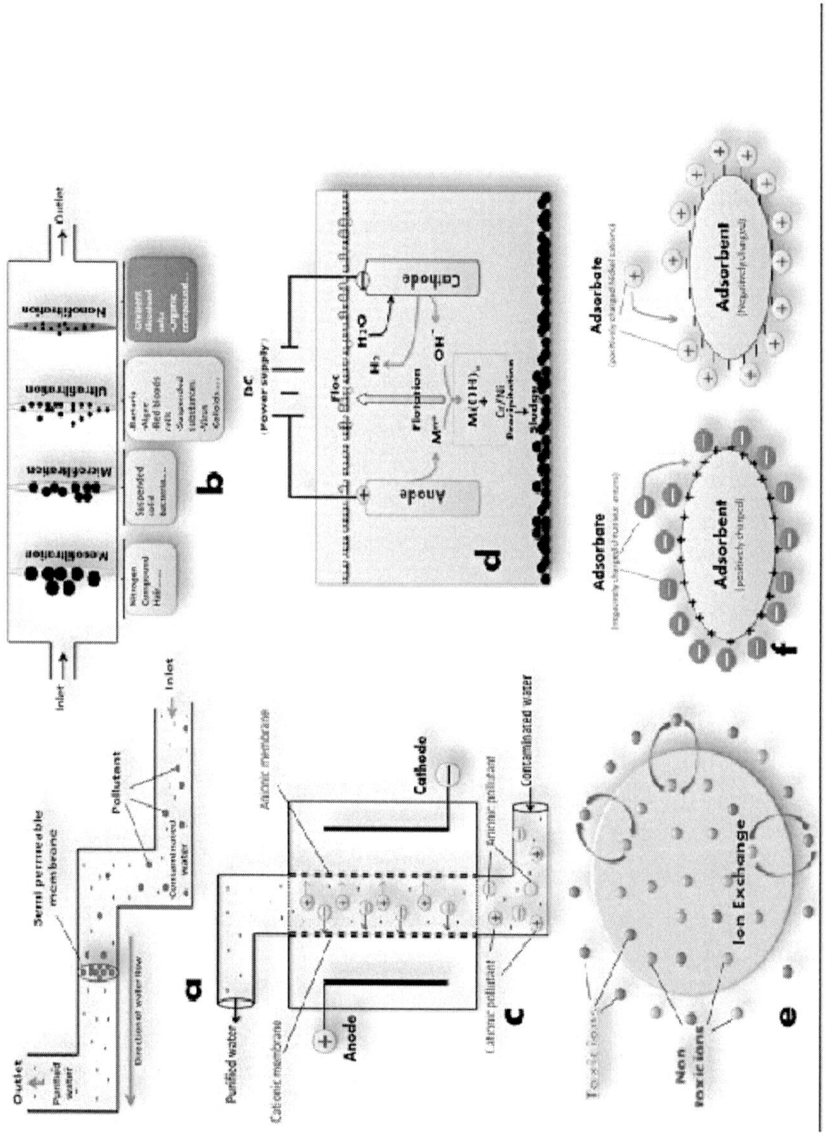

Fig 2: Different Types of Techniques Used in Cr-VI Removal. [21, 30]

6. DEVELOPMENT OF CONCEPTUAL METHODOLOGY SUITABLE FOR MINING AREAS

The techniques used before have their pros and cons. Keeping in view all the disadvantages and advantages, we have hypothesized a cost-effective and environmentally feasible hybrid-type process by combining the following methods as shown in the below flow diagram [Fig 3]:

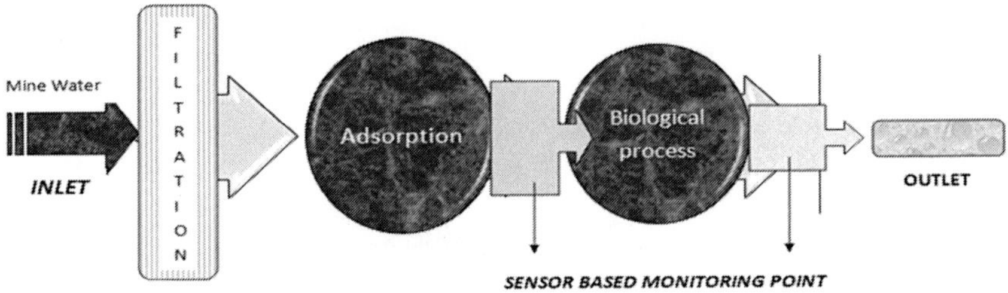

Fig: 3 A hybrid water treatment system with sensor-based monitoring system: Flow Chart

Membrane Filtration: Water discharged from the mine will directly undergo a filtration method for which an appropriate filter will be chosen for its removal efficiency.

Adsorption: The pre-treated water will then enter another system for treatment through adsorption. We have studied lots of adsorbents and their efficiency from the above literature. By experimentation, we will use an adsorbent which will be environmentally friendly as well as show great removal efficiency.

Constructed Wetland: Above discussions depicted that the specific types of plants have significant absorbing capacities of heavy metals present in the wastewater. We will allow the water to undergo treatment through the biological process in the next system. As removal potential generally reduces after a few hours of adsorption, plants in the constructed wetland will strengthen their removal capacity. Appropriate plants will be chosen for a constructed wetland due to their easy availability, feasibility and removal capacity.

We expect that Sensor Based Monitoring will be much more helpful as it will help monitor a large amount of water discharged from mines. After every treatment system, a sensor will be put in to monitor its removal rate individually. We will construct a prototype of the hypothesized Cr-VI treatment plant and test this in the laboratory. After getting an optimized result, we will test the system case study mine areas.

7. CONCLUSION

In the last decade, extensive research has been conducted to investigate the importance of contaminated metals from water. Bioremediation is a general expression for several ways in which plants remediate sites by removing pollutants from the water as it stabilises metal contaminants by acting as a filter. Given the above facts, it is worth using plant species which are easily available and integrating them with adsorbents to strengthen the removing capacity and eliminate Cr-VI from the mine water. The main advantages of this designed hybrid system are an environment-friendly, cost-effective and efficient Cr-VI removing process.

REFERENCES

1. Unceta N, Séby F, Malherbe J, Donard OF. Chromium speciation in solid matrices and regulation: a review. Anal Bioanal Chem. 2010 https://pubmed.ncbi.nlm.nih.gov/20099060/
2. Rai D, Eary LE, Zachara JM. Environmental chemistry of Chromium. Sci Total Environ. 1989Oct1. https://pubmed.ncbi.nlm.nih.gov/2602932/
3. Bokare A.D., Choi W. Advanced Oxidation Process Based on the Cr-III/Cr-VI Redox Cycle. Environ. Sci. Technol. 2011. https://pubs.acs.org/doi/abs/10.1021/es2021704
4. Involvement of calcium, reactive oxygen species, and ATP in hexavalent chromium-induced damage in red blood cells. *Zhang R, Xiang Y, Ran Q, Deng X, Xiao Y, Xiang L, Li ZCell Physiol Biochem. 2014; 34(5):1780-91* https://pubmed.ncbi.nlm.nih.gov/25427846/
5. Toxic and genotoxic effects of hexavalent Chromium in the environment and its bioremediation strategies. *Mishra S, Bharagava RNJ Environ Sci Health C Environ Carcinog Ecotoxicol Rev. 2016; 34(1):1-32* https://pubmed.ncbi.nlm.nih.gov/26398402/
6. Remediation of hexavalent chromium contaminated water through zero-valent iron nanoparticles and effects on tomato plant growth performance. Brasili E, Bavasso I, Petruccelli V, Vilardi G, Valletta A, Dal Bosco C, Gentili A, Pasqua G, Di Palma LSci Rep. 2020 Feb 5; 10(1):1920

7. Chromium(VI) sorption efficiency of acid-activated banana peel over organo-montmorillonite in aqueous solutions. *Ashraf A, Bibi I, Niazi NK, Ok YS, Murtaza G, Shahid M, Kunhikrishnan A, Li D, Mahmood Tint J Phytoremediation. 2017 Jul 3;* https://pubmed.ncbi.nlm.nih.gov/27849143/
8. Origin of hexavalent Chromium in groundwater: The example of Sarigkiol Basin, Northern Greece. Kazakis N, Kantiranis N, Kalaitzidou K, Kaprara E, Mitrakas M, Frei R, Vargemezis G, Tsourlos P, Zouboulis A, Filippidis ASci Total Environ. 2017 Sep 1; 593-https://pubmed.ncbi.nlm.nih.gov/28360005/
9. Yang Y, Ma H, Chen X, Zhu C, Li X. Effect of incineration temperature on chromium speciation in real chromium-rich tannery sludge under air atmosphere. Environ Res. 2020 Apr. https://pubmed.ncbi.nlm.nih.gov/32028182/
10. Microbial reduction fate of Chromium (Cr) in aqueous solution by mixed bacterial consortium. Ma L, Xu J, Chen N, Li M, Feng CEcotoxicol Environ Saf. 2019 Apr 15; 170():763770 https://pubmed.ncbi.nlm.nih.gov/30583287/
11. Koleli N., Demir A. Environmental Materials and Waste. Academic Press; London, UK: 2016. Chromite; pp. 245–263. https://www.ncbi.nlm.nih.gov/pmc/articles/PMC7432837/
12. Sanchez-Segado S., Makanyire T., Escudero-Castejon L., Hara Y., Jha A. Reclamation of reactive metal oxides from complex minerals using alkali roasting and leaching—An improved approach to process engineering. *Green Chem.* 2015 https://pubs.rsc.org/en/content/articlelanding/2015/gc/c4gc02360a
13. Katsoyiannis I.A., Xanthopoulou M., Zouboulis A.I. Cr-VI Femoval from Ground Waters by Ferrous Iron Redox-Assisted Coagulation in a Continuous Treatment Unit Comprising a Plug Flow Pipe Reactor and Downflow Sand Filtration. *Appl. Sci.* 2020 https://www.mdpi.com/2076-3417/10/3/802
14. Shi L., Zhang X., Chen Z. Removal of Chromium (VI) from wastewater using bentonite- supported nanoscale zero-valent iron. *WaterRes.* 2011. https://www.ncbi.nlm.nih.gov/pmc/articles/PMC8537176/
15. Plummer S., Gorman C., Henrie T., Shimabuku K., Thompson R., Seidel C. Optimizing strong-base anion exchange O&M costs for hexavalent chromium treatment. *Water Res.* 2018. https://pubmed.ncbi.nlm.nih.gov/29709799/
16. Dermentzis K., Christophoridis A., Valsamidou E., Lazaridou A., Kokkinos N. Removal of hexavalent Chromium from electroplating

wastewater by electro-coagulation with iron electrodes. *Glob. NESTJ.* 2011. https://www.cabdirect.org/cabdirect/abstract/20123125171
17. Sukinda Chromite Mine goes organic to tackle the Hexavalent Chromium problem, Bhubaneswar, June 24, 2011, https://www.tatasteel.com/media/newsroom/press-releases/india/2011/sukinda-chromite-mine-goes-organic-to-tackle-the-hexavalent-chromium-problem/
18. Barrera-Díaz CE, Lugo-Lugo V, Bilyeu B. A review of chemical, electrochemical and biological methods for aqueous Cr-VI reduction. J Hazard Mater. 2012 Jul https://pubmed.ncbi.nlm.nih.gov/22608208/
19. https://www.researchgate.net/publication/51499982_Chromium_in_Drinking_Water_Sources_Metabolism_and_Cancer_Risks, accessed on 18th July, 2022.
20. Kimbrough, David & Cohen, Yoram & Winer, Arthur & Creelman, Lynn & Mabuni, Clayton. (1999). A Critical Assessment of Chromium in the Environment. Critical Reviews in Environmental Science and Technology Critical Reviews Environmental Science and Technology, https://www.tandfonline.com/doi/abs/10.1080/10643389991259164
21. Shalenie P. den Braver-Sewradj, Jan van Benthem, Yvonne C.M. Staal, Janine Ezendam, Aldert H. Piersma, Ellen V.S. Hessel, Occupational exposure to hexavalent Chromium. Part II. Hazard assessment of carcinogenic effects, Regulatory Toxicology and Pharmacology, Volume 126, 2021 https://www.sciencedirect.com/science/article/pii/S0273230021001860
22. Debabrata Pradhan, Lala Behari Sukla, Matthew Sawyer, Pattanathu K.S.M. Rahman, Recent bioreduction of hexavalent Chromium in wastewater treatment: A review, https://pure.port.ac.uk/ws/portalfiles/portal/12113465/Recent_bioreduction_of_hexavalent_chromium.pdf
23. https://www.businesshumanrights.org/en/latest-news/blacksmith-institute-reports-on-top-10-worst-polluted-places-in-the-world-financial-times-article/, accessed on 17th August 2022
24. Haripriya Mishra and Himanshu Bhusan Sahu, Environmental Scenario of Chromite Mining at Sukinda Valley – A Review, International Journal of Environmental Engineering and Management, ISSN 2231-1319, Volume 4, Number 4 (2013), pp. 287-292
25. N-SITU remediation of heavy metals using sulfur-based treatment

technologies, Jim Jacobs, Roy L. Hardison, and Jim V. Rouse.

26. Renitta Jobby, Pamela Jha, Anoop Kumar Yadav, Nitin Desai, Biosorption and biotransformation of hexavalent Chromium [Cr-VI]: A comprehensive review, Chemosphere, Volume 207, 2018.
27. Vinay Kumar, S.K. Dwivedi, A review on accessible techniques for removal of hexavalent Chromium and divalent Nickel from industrial wastewater: Recent research and future outlook, Journal of Cleaner Production, Volume 295, 2021. https://www.sciencedirect.com/science/article/abs/pii/S0959652621004492
28. Chen, Yanliang & Zhao, L. & Wei, Y.-Z & He, L.-F & Tang, F.-D. (2015). Adsorption characteristics of thorium on silica-based anion exchange resins.
29. Garba, M.D., Usman, M., Mazumder, M.A.J. *et al.* Complexing agents for metal removal using ultrafiltration membranes: a review. *EnvironChemLett* (2019). Complexing agents for metal removal using ultrafiltration membranes: a review | SpringerLink.
30. Tortora, F., Innocenzi, V., Prisciandaro, M. *et al.* Heavy Metal Removal from Liquid Wastes by Using Micellar-Enhanced Ultrafiltration. *WaterAirSoil Pollut* **227,** 240 (2016). https://link.springer.com/article/10.1007/s11270-016-2935-7#citeas
31. A. Otero-Fernández, J.A. Otero, A. Maroto, J. Carmona, L. Palacio, P. Prádanos, A. Hernández, Concentration-polarization in nanofiltration of low concentration Cr VI aqueous solutions. Effect of operative conditions on retention, Journal of Cleaner Production, Volume 150, 2017.
32. Comparative study of the removal of nickel(II) and chromium(VI) heavy metals from metal plating wastewater by two nanofiltration membranes: Desalination and Water Treatment: Vol 57, No 46.
33. Mahendra S. Gaikwad, Chandrajit Balomajumder, Simultaneous rejection of Chromium (VI) and fluoride [Cr-VI and F] by nanofiltration: Membranes characterizations and estimations of membrane transport parameters by CFSK model, Journal of Environmental Chemical Engineering, Volume 5, Issue 1, 2017.
34. Soroosh Mortazavian, Ali Saber, Jaeyoung Hong, Jee-Hwan Bae, Dongwon Chun, Nicolas Wong, Daniel Gerrity, Jacimaria Batista, Kwang J. Kim, Jaeyun Moon, Synthesis, characterization, and kinetic study of activated carbon modified by polysulfide rubber coating for aqueous hexavalent chromium removal, Journal of Industrial and Engineering Chemistry, Volume 69, 2019.
35. Kumar, Paritosh & Kaur, Ravinder & Defo, Celestin & Kumar,

Prakash. (2020). Plant, microbe, and media chromium removal efficiency in experimental VSSF constructed wetlands under monocropped and co-cropped conditions. Environmental Science and Pollution Research, volume 27, pages 2071–2086 (2020)
36. You, Shao-Hong & Zhang, Xue-Hong & Liu, Jie & Zhu, Yinian & Gu, Chen. (2014). Feasibility of constructed wetland planted with Leersia hexandra Swartz for removing Cr, Cu and Ni from electroplating wastewater. Environmental technology. 35. 187-94. 10.1080/09593330.2013.822006.
37. Guoqi Lian, Bing Wang, Xinqing Lee, Ling Li, Taoze Liu, Wenqiang Lyu, Enhanced removal of hexavalent Chromium by engineered biochar composite fabricated from phosphogypsum and distillers grains, Science of The Total Environment, Volume 697, 2019.
38. Guoqi Lian, Bing Wang, Xinqing Lee, Ling Li, Taoze Liu, Wenqiang Lyu, Enhanced removal of hexavalent Chromium by engineered biochar composite fabricated from phosphogypsum and distillers grains, Science of The Total Environment, Volume 697, 2019.
39. Rod, Kenton, Schuyler, Kimberly A., & Hall, Stephen H. *Hexavalent chromium sensor for real-time In situ measurement of groundwater contamination - 15433*. United States.
40. https://cfpub.epa.gov/ncer_abstracts/index.cfm/fuseaction/display.abstractDetail/abstract_id/1721/report/0 accessed on 20th August, 2022.
41. Sverre Langård, Max Costa, Chapter 33 - Chromium, Editor(s): Gunnar F. Nordberg, Bruce A. Fowler, Monica Nordberg, Handbook on the Toxicology of Metals (Fourth Edition), Academic Press, 2015.
42. Mishra, Haripriya & Sahu, Himanshu. (2013). Environmental Scenario of Chromite Mining at Sukinda Valley A Review, 287292.

CHAPTER 7

SOFT ACTUATOR-BASED DRUG DELIVERY SYSTEM

MARIATUL RAWDHAH AHMAD FUAAD[1], MOHAMMED NAZIBUL HASAN[2], MOHAMED SULTAN MOHAMED ALI[1,3]

[1]Faculty of Electrical Engineering, Universiti Teknologi Malaysia, 81310 UTM Johor Bahru, Johor, Malaysia;
[2]Division of Solid-State Electronics, Department of Electrical Engineering, Uppsala University, SE-75103, Uppsala, Sweden;
[3]Department of Electrical Engineering, College of Engineering, Qatar University, Doha, Qatar

ABSTRACT

This study aims to explore the impact of technological advancements on drug delivery technologies, mainly focusing on using soft actuators to develop microfluidic systems for drug delivery. The discussion centres on the potential of soft actuators to enable the controlled release of therapeutics and respond to stimuli such as temperature. The study overviews previous soft actuation technologies such as shape memory polymers (SMP) and thermo-pneumatic actuators. In addition, the latest soft actuation technology that combines electrostatic and hydraulic actuation, resulting in fluid-amplified dielectric elastomer actuators (DEA), was also reviewed. The study also describes the amplification displacement of fluid-amplified DEA and its functioning in microfluidic systems. The developed actuator can provide displacement amplification of ~4×, while the micropump can achieve flow rates of up to ~2200 μl/min. The advancements discussed in this chapter provide a foundation for further exploration and development in this field and the potential for future innovations in drug delivery technology.

Keywords: *Soft actuator; drug delivery, shape memory polymer, dielectric elastomer*

1. INTRODUCTION

The COVID-19 pandemic has caused a significant strain on healthcare systems, with hospitals becoming overwhelmed with in-patients. In this context, drug delivery systems can be particularly useful in providing access to medications for out-patients. These systems allow for minimal administration and can minimise the need for patients to visit hospitals or clinics, thereby reducing the burden on the healthcare system and protecting patients from potential exposure to the virus. Additionally, drug delivery systems can improve treatment outcomes by ensuring patients receive the appropriate medication dosage at the appropriate intervals. In summary, drug delivery systems can improve access to medicine and enhance treatment effectiveness during the COVID-19 pandemic.

The therapeutics landscape evolution has led to the development of various drug delivery technologies that enhance the delivery of pharmaceutical products to their target site. One major challenge in drug delivery is formulating systems with controlled release. The drug's minimum effective and maximum therapeutic concentrations can vary from patient to patient and may differ for each drug [1]. Microfluidic technologies can be used to develop drug delivery systems that provide controlled release of various therapeutics, including small molecules, proteins, peptides, nucleic acids, live cells, and monoclonal antibodies (mAbs) [2]. The tiny channels and tubes in microfluidic devices can precisely control the drug's flow and dosage, enabling the delivery of the minimum effective concentration to the target site while avoiding toxic concentrations [3]. Additionally, microfluidic devices can be designed to release the drug in response to certain stimuli, such as changes in pH or temperature, which can further enhance the control of drug delivery. Overall, microfluidic technology has the potential to improve the effectiveness and safety of drug delivery systems significantly.

Micropumps are small pumps that utilise micro-electro-mechanical systems (MEMS) technology to move small volumes of fluids. They are often used in conjunction with microfluidic devices, which are systems containing microscale channels or tubes that allow for the flow of fluids. The compact size and precise control of micropumps make them well-suited for use in microfluidic systems, where they can accurately regulate the flow of fluids. Shape Memory Alloy, an intelligent material, has been adopted in various MEMS devices [4, 5]. However, the rigid nature of SMA limits its application range. Micropumps that use shape-memory polymer (SMP), thermo-pneumatics and dielectric elastomers soft actuators as the driving force are utilised in various applications, for instance, the drug delivery system, chemical synthesis, and environmental monitoring [6-9]. This chapter reviews the different actuation mechanisms used in drug delivery systems, including SMP, thermo-pneumatic, and dielectric elastomers. Furthermore, the latest technology for fluid-amplified DEA in micropumps is examined. Finally, the amplification displacement of the fluid-amplified DEA and its functioning within the micropump system are discussed in detail.

2. SOFT-BASED ACTUATORS FOR DRUG DELIVERY SYSTEMS

This section focuses on the prominent soft actuation mechanisms that are used in drug delivery systems, including SMP, thermo-pneumatic materials, and dielectric elastomers. These mechanisms offer the ability to control the drug release from a device in a precise and responsive manner.

2.1 Shape Memory Polymer

SMP-utilised drug delivery has been widely adopted for handling various therapeutics, including small molecules and new-generation therapeutics. These SMP drug delivery devices exhibit excellent features, like high drug loading [10], activated wirelessly [11] and two-way actuation [12]. Previous research has reported using SMP in drug-delivery devices. However, several design challenges exist, such as their incompatibility with bulk-SMP and the need to blend them with fillers [13]. Additionally, using carbon nanotubes as fillers in SMP composites is impractical for implantable devices [14, 15], negatively impacting their performance. Thus, innovative design techniques are necessary to address these limitations. Zainal et al. has developed an implantable drug delivery device based on an SMP/polyimide (PI) laminate actuator [16], as illustrated in **Figure 1a**. The device prototype incorporates a heater, which is a planar LC (inductor-capacitor) resonant circuit to regulate the SMP material temperature.

When an AC magnetic field that matches the resonant frequency of an LC circuit is applied, the energy from the field causes the LC circuit to oscillate at a high amplitude, resulting in the heating of the circuit due to the induced electromotive force. The SMP actuator is affixed to the heater, constructed from a copper-clad polyimide (Cu-clad PI) sheet, forming an

SMP/PI structure. The Cu-clad PI is both a heat source and a stress layer, providing deformation through the bimorph principle. In addition, the device utilises the SMP's shape memory effect, allowing easy deformation when exposed to temperatures above the glass transition temperature. This device uses the SMP to seal the drug reservoir after it is bonded to the device, and the drug administration is through a small hole installed in the reservoir. The LC resonant circuit, functioning as a heater, activates the SMP actuator and dispenses the drug. The simulation results of the device design, obtained using the finite element tool COMSOL Multiphysics™, indicate that the design provides ample space between the actuator and reservoir during actuation.

2.2 Thermo-pneumatic

Micropumps and micromixers have grown significantly in microfluidics as they are popular research subjects. These devices are frequently used in biomedical systems, such as therapeutic implant devices [17] and lab-on-chip systems [18], due to their ability to precisely control fluid dosage and manipulate fluids within small-scale geometries. Various actuation mechanisms have been developed, including those for refractory epilepsy treatment [19], pain management [20], controlled growth factor delivery [21], and in-vitro diabetic injection [22] to achieve compatibility with clinical applications. These mechanisms contrast with other actuation techniques that have been developed, such as those based on electromagnetic [23, 24], piezoelectric [25, 26], and pneumatic principles [27, 28]. A thermo-pneumatic actuation is a viable option for biomedical applications due to its low operating voltage and eliminating the need for additional peripheral driving equipment.

A thermo-pneumatic micropump utilises a membrane displacement resulting from the air expansion and contraction in response to variations in temperature within the heating region. A study presented an RF-powered wireless thermo-pneumatic micropump that is controlled by adjusting the frequency of the external magnetic field [29] (illustrated in **Figure 1c**). The device was designed without moving parts, improving reliability and durability during pumping operations. In addition, the ability to wirelessly adjust the flow rate with the developed micropump was proven experimentally, validating the feasibility of the actuation principle of RF thermo-pneumatic. The micropump design comprises a PDMS-made outlet hole, loading reservoir and heating chamber. The liquid sample is transferred from the loading reservoir to the outlet port via the microchannel. A diffuser in the microchannel prevents fluids from overflowing into the heating chamber. This micropump uses a mechanism that allows it to move the liquid in one direction without using mechanical moving parts or continuous liquid intake, thus preventing any leakage from the diffuser during the pumping process. A cover lid of 2mm thickness encloses the fluid-directing channel to minimize air leakage from the heating chamber to the adjacent area.

Another application of thermo-pneumatic technology can also be found in micromixers [30-33]. Researchers have developed a passive, wirelessly controlled thermo-pneumatic micromixer [34] to address challenges associated with implantable drug delivery devices using micromixers (refer to **Figure 1b**). The device utilises an actuation method through radio frequency magnetic fields. It can selectively operate multiple heaters, which is crucial for new applications such as the selective delivery of various drugs at specific concentrations for multiple clinical purposes. The micromixer comprises two loading reservoirs, two micro diffuser elements, two air-heating chambers, two inductor-capacitor (LC) wireless heaters, an outlet hole, and a zigzag micromixing element. These components are assembled to form a device that can mix liquid on a small scale and control the heating of the liquid with wireless heaters using the LC circuit and air-heating chambers. The device can regulate the mixing ratio precisely. Its planar geometry can be fabricated utilising non-sterile fabrication processes, making it a cost-effective solution for biomedical applications such as localised drug delivery and cell culturing.

2.3 Dielectric Elastomer

Dielectric Elastomer Actuators (DEA), an Electroactive Polymers (EAP) category, possess large deformability and fast response times. These characteristics result from low power consumption, making them a viable alternative to traditional actuation methods. DEAs have a good energy density similar to human muscles and high strain potential with a remarkable force-to-weight ratio. A DEA comprises a pair of electrodes on either side of a dielectric elastomer, generating compressive electrostatic stress resulting in strain and surface expansion during actuation [35].

Ghazali et al. [36] demonstrated the DEA actuation and micropump integration (**Figure 1d**). The DEA performance was evaluated by experimenting with various DEA membrane thicknesses and sizes. The DEA was designed to function as a diffuser micropump and was constructed using VHB film, PDMS, and carbon powder. DEA micropump functions are based on the same principle as an electrostatically actuated micropump using the flexible actuator membrane's bending motion to control the pump chamber's fluid flow. The DEA micro pump is a cost-effective alternative to other micropumps, as it is made of biocompatible polymer-based materials and can prevent backflow in the pump chamber.

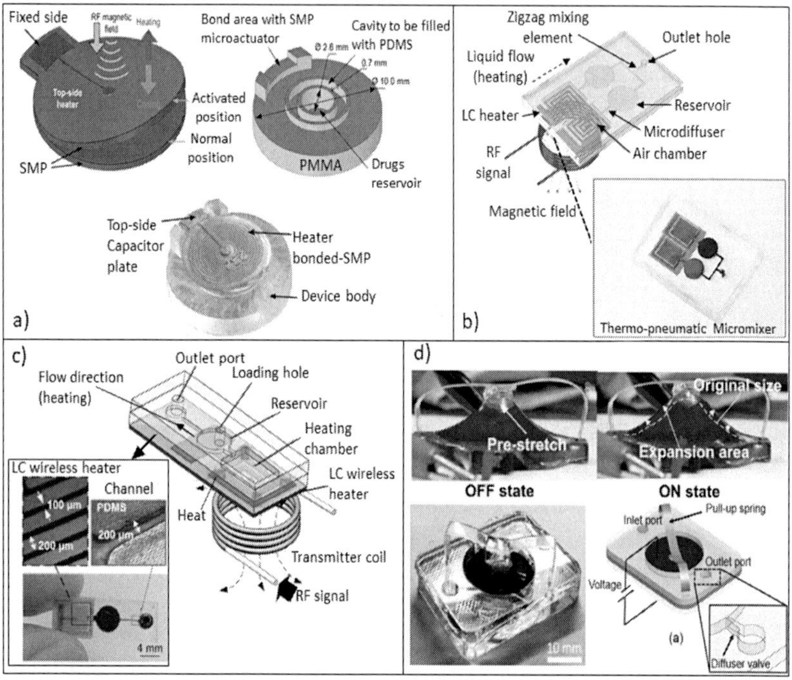

Figure 1 a) SMP-based drug delivery. Reproduced with permission from Ref. [14]. Copyright 2017, Springer Nature. b) Thermo-pneumatic micromixer. Reproduced with permission from Ref. [32]. Copyright 2017, IEEE. c) Thermo-pneumatic micropump. Reproduced with permission from Ref. [27]. Copyright 2015, Elsevier. d) DEA micropump. Reproduced with permission from Ref. [34]. Copyright 2017, Elsevier

2.4 Fluid-amplified DE

Acome et al. [37] first introduced the fluid-amplified DEA technology in 2018, an innovative approach that combines the best features of DEA and fluid-driven soft actuator technologies while also addressing DEA's limitations. It offers a significant advantage in displacement and versatility because it can perform all basic actuation modes due to the addition of dielectric fluid, resulting in increased removal. The fluid-amplified DEA consists of a dielectric fluid-filled elastomeric shell between two opposing electrodes. The high voltage applied across the electrodes causes a potential difference, creating compressive electrostatic forces (also known as Maxwell stress) between them. Hydraulic pressure inside the elastomer shell is linked to Maxwell pressure, *P*, which is defined as:

$$P \propto \varepsilon E^2$$

Where *E* is the applied electric field, and ε is the dielectric permittivity of the elastomer or fluid [38]. As the voltage increases, the actuation strain of the elastomer or fluid rises in proportion to the applied electric field, *E*. When the voltage surpasses a certain threshold, the pull-in transition, also known as zipping, happens as the increase in electrostatic force becomes more significant than the mechanical restoring force.

As previously discussed, there have been efforts to incorporate DEA in micropump applications [39]. However, due to the high risk of dielectric breakdown damage that DEA are prone to, it presents an opportunity to implement fluid-amplified DEA in micropump applications. In addition, fluid-amplified DEA is more resilient to high voltage, making them a more suitable option for micropump applications. To the best of the author's knowledge, the fluid-amplified DEA implementation in microfluidics has yet to be studied. The micropump in this study was fabricated using a low-cost method similar to that of fluid-amplified DEA. The micropump design includes four main components: the pump chamber, actuator chamber, inlet flap, and outlet flap, all made of polydimethylsiloxane (PDMS) and Ecoflex (illustrated in **Figure 2**).

These components were fabricated using a 3D-printing mould and casting process. The flaps were designed to prevent fluid backflow and allow only one flow direction. The micropump's membrane was designed to act as a diaphragm, causing pressure oscillation in the pump chamber and permitting fluid displacement. The micropump's operation can be classified into supply and pump modes. Low pressure in the pump chamber causes the inlet flap to be open and draw fluid in when the pump is in supply mode. However, when the pump is in pump mode, high pressure in the chamber causes the fluid to be expelled through the outlet flap. The present study evaluated the performance and characteristics of a micropump that incorporated fluid-amplified DEA technology. The fabricated device's loading capacity fluid was determined by pre-priming it with deionized water. This process, known as pre-priming, involves filling the pump and supply line with deionised water and expelling any air that may be present in the passageways.

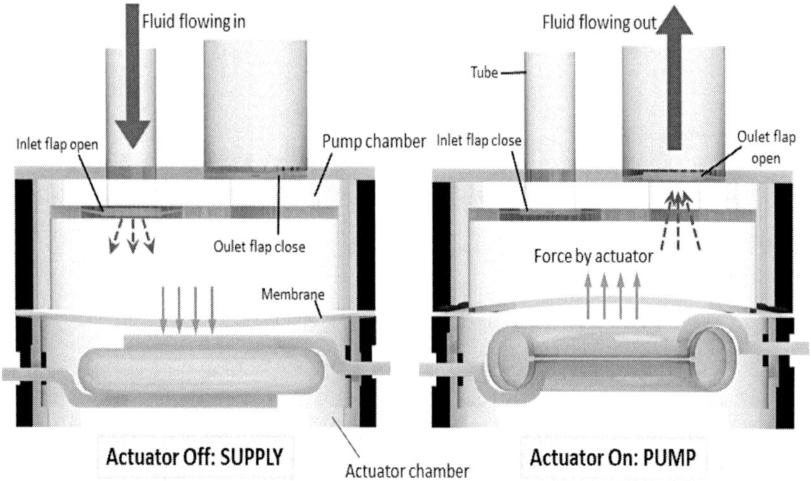

Figure 2 Fluid-amplified DEA in micropump mechanism

As illustrated in Figure 3a, the actuator amplification plays a crucial role in the micropump's pumping mechanism. This amplification is defined as out-of-plane displacement of the fluid-amplified DEA caused by the electrodes zipping due to the Maxwell stress acting on the displaced dielectric fluid from between the electrodes to the outer ring area (as indicated in equation 1). A laser displacement sensor was utilised to record the movement at the centre (electrode) and outer ring to accurately measure the actuator displacement. The displacement vs time graph in **Figure 3b** clearly shows the amplification of the fluid-amplified DEA. The results demonstrate that the displacement at the outer ring was approximately four times greater than the displacement at the centre due to the soft and elastic structure of the fluid-amplified DEA.

Figure 4a demonstrates the water level changes that occurred due to activating the fluid-amplified DEA for three minutes, providing qualitative evidence of the device's pumping capabilities. **Figure 4b** shows that the flow rate increases as the operating frequency increases, peaking at 2304 μL/min within the 0.1 to 0.25 Hz range. However, as the frequency rises, the flow rate decreases, indicating that the actuator does not respond at frequencies higher than 0.25 Hz.

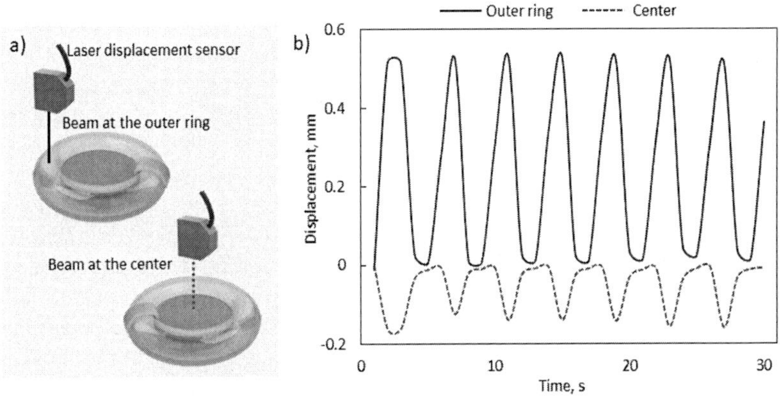

Figure 3 a) Experimental setup and b) amplification of fluid-amplified DEA

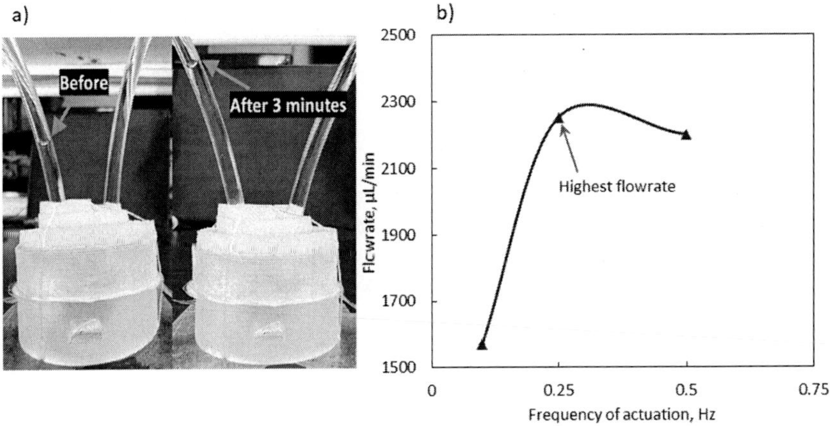

Figure 4 a) Fluid-amplified DEA micropump device and b) flow rate at three actuation frequencies.

3. SUMMARY & CONCLUSION

Realising soft-based MEMS drug delivery devices with proper fabrication and function techniques for clinical use is challenging. MEMS are a rapidly growing technology for drug delivery because they can be designed to deliver drugs at a special rate, at a specific time, and at a specific location in the body. In this chapter, we present four actuation mechanisms: SMP, thermo-pneumatic, DEA, and fluid-amplified DEA, and discuss their drug delivery application's potential due to their excellent features. The SMP technique is a promising technology for drug delivery. It allows for memorising the interchangeable shape and offers high elastic deformation and structural flexibility producing large force and displacement, making them usable for micropump and micromixer applications. However, SMPs have limitations, such as low operational frequency and thermal stability, limiting their use in some applications. Meanwhile, thermo-pneumatic is widely used for micropump/micromixer, offering bidirectional motion, high power-to-weight ratio and high displacement. Based on the thermal expansion and contraction principle, this technology allows pressure and flow rate control for drug delivery. However, it is limited by its low-frequency operation and the need for high power consumption. The DEA technique provides a significant deformability degree, high actuation strain (> 100%), and excellent electromechanical performance, allowing a significant flow rate in the drug delivery system. Nonetheless, DEAs are limited by their low durability and poor reliability.

Recently developed technology, such as the fluid-amplified DEA technique, has been utilised to advance its integration into micropump systems. The technique's beneficial features have been leveraged to achieve this progress. The fluid-amplified DEA technique is based on the principle of electro-hydrostatic actuation; it allows for significant displacement and high force. However, the fluid-amplified DEA is still in the early development stage, and further research is needed to improve its reliability and durability. The potential of these actuation mechanisms has been demonstrated through their practical application in various drug delivery systems, such as micropumps and micromixers. The continued advancements in these emerging technologies can lead to further breakthroughs and improvements in other healthcare systems utilising MEMS technology. Other soft actuators that could potentially used for achieving large actuation are pneumatic type actuators [40, 41].

REFERENCES

[1] L. Shargel, B. Andrew, and S. Wu-Pong, *Applied biopharmaceutics & pharmacokinetics*. Appleton & Lange Stamford, 1999.

[2] A. M. Vargason, A. C. Anselmo, and S. Mitragotri, "The evolution of commercial drug delivery technologies," *Nature biomedical engineering,* vol. 5, no. 9, pp. 951-967, 2021.

[3] S. Adepu and S. Ramakrishna, "Controlled drug delivery systems: current status and future directions," *Molecules,* vol. 26, no. 19, p. 5905, 2021.

[4] A. AbuZaiter, M. Nafea, A. A. M. Faudzi, S. Kazi, and M. S. M. Ali, "Thermomechanical behaviour of bulk NiTi shape-memory-

alloy microactuators based on bimorph actuation," *Microsystem Technologies,* vol. 22, no. 8, pp. 2125-2131, 2016.
[5] M. R. A. Kadir, D. E. O. Dewi, M. N. Jamaludin, M. Nafea, and M. S. M. Ali, "A multi-segmented shape memory alloy-based actuator system for endoscopic applications," *Sensors and Actuators A: Physical,* vol. 296, pp. 92-100, 2019.
[6] A. Saini, D. Ahmad, and K. Patra, "Electromechanical performance analysis of inflated dielectric elastomer membrane for micro pump applications," in *Electroactive Polymer Actuators and Devices (EAPAD) 2016*, 2016, vol. 9798: SPIE, pp. 180-186.
[7] M. Ebara, K. Uto, N. Idota, J. M. Hoffman, and T. Aoyagi, "Rewritable and shape-memory soft matter with dynamically tunable microchannel geometry in a biological temperature range," *Soft Matter,* vol. 9, no. 11, pp. 3074-3080, 2013.
[8] P. S. Chee, M. Nafea, P. L. Leow, and M. S. M. Ali, "Thermal analysis of wirelessly powered thermo-pneumatic micropump based on planar LC circuit," *Journal of Mechanical Science and Technology,* vol. 30, no. 6, pp. 2659-2665, 2016.
[9] F. Ghazali, M. Hasan, T. Rehman, M. Nafea, M. S. Mohamed Ali, and K. Takahata, "MEMS actuators for biomedical applications: a review," *Journal of Micromechanics and Microengineering,* vol. 30, pp. 073001-073020, 05/28 2020, DoI: 10.1088/1361-6439/ab8832.
[10] K. Cai *et al.*, "Dimeric drug polymeric nanoparticles with exceptionally high drug loading and quantitative loading efficiency," *Journal of the American Chemical Society,* vol. 137, no. 10, pp. 3458-3461, 2015.
[11] E. Chappel, "Implantable drug delivery devices," in *Drug Delivery Devices and Therapeutic Systems*: Elsevier, 2021, pp. 129-156.
[12] W. Zhao, L. Liu, F. Zhang, J. Leng, and Y. Liu, "Shape memory polymers and their composites in biomedical applications," *Materials Science and Engineering: C,* vol. 97, pp. 864-883, 2019.
[13] Y. Wang, R. Zhao, S. Wang, Z. Liu, and R. Tang, "In vivo dual-targeted chemotherapy of drug resistant cancer by rationally designed nanocarrier," *Biomaterials,* vol. 75, pp. 71-81, 2016.
[14] F.-P. Du *et al.*, "Electroactive shape memory polymer based on optimized multi-walled carbon nanotubes/polyvinyl alcohol nanocomposites," *Composites Part B: Engineering,* vol. 68, pp. 170-175, 2015.

[15] H. Lu, Y. Yao, and L. Lin, "Carbon-based reinforcement in shape-memory polymer composite for electrical actuation," *Pigment & Resin Technology,* vol. 43, no. 1, pp. 26-34, 2014.
[16] M. Zainal, A. Ahmad, and M. M. Ali, "Frequency-controlled wireless shape memory polymer microactuator for drug delivery application," *Biomedical microdevices,* vol. 19, no. 1, p. 8, 2017.
[17] W. Whyte *et al.*, "Dynamic actuation enhances transport and extends therapeutic lifespan in an implantable drug delivery platform," *Nature Communications,* vol. 13, no. 1, pp. 1-17, 2022.
[18] A. Maurice, J. Theisen, and J.-C. P. Gabriel, "Microfluidic lab-on-chip advances for liquid–liquid extraction process studies," *Current Opinion in Colloid & Interface Science,* vol. 46, pp. 20-35, 2020.
[19] M. A. Sayeed, S. P. Mohanty, E. Kougianos, and H. P. Zaveri, "An IoT-based drug delivery system for refractory epilepsy," in *2019 IEEE International Conference on Consumer Electronics (ICCE)*, 2019: IEEE, pp. 1-4.
[20] H. Gensler, R. Sheybani, P.-Y. Li, R. L. Mann, and E. Meng, "An implantable MEMS micropump system for drug delivery in small animals," *Biomedical microdevices,* vol. 14, no. 3, pp. 483-496, 2012.
[21] Z. Wang, Z. Wang, W. W. Lu, W. Zhen, D. Yang, and S. Peng, "Novel biomaterial strategies for controlled growth factor delivery for biomedical applications," *NPG Asia Materials,* vol. 9, no. 10, pp. e435-e435, 2017.
[22] B. Yan *et al.*, "Battery-free implantable insulin micropump operating at transcutaneously radio frequency-transmittable power," *Medical Devices & Sensors,* vol. 2, no. 5-6, p. e10055, 2019.
[23] V. H. Le *et al.*, "A soft-magnet-based drug-delivery module for active locomotive intestinal capsule endoscopy using an electromagnetic actuation system," *Sensors and Actuators A: Physical,* vol. 243, pp. 81-89, 2016.
[24] R. R. Gidde, P. M. Pawar, B. P. Ronge, and V. P. Dhamgaye, "Design optimization of an electromagnetic actuation based valveless micropump for drug delivery application," *Microsystem Technologies,* vol. 25, no. 2, pp. 509-519, 2019.
[25] K. Srinivasa Rao, M. Hamza, P. Ashok Kumar, and K. Girija Sravani, "Design and optimization of MEMS based piezoelectric actuator for drug delivery systems," *Microsystem Technologies,* vol. 26, no. 5, pp. 1671-1679, 2020.

[26] M. Nafea, A. Nawabjan, and M. S. M. Ali, "A wirelessly-controlled piezoelectric microvalve for regulated drug delivery," *Sensors and Actuators A: Physical,* vol. 279, pp. 191-203, 2018.
[27] Y.-S. Chen, C. P.-K. Lai, C. Chen, and G.-B. Lee, "Isolation and recovery of extracellular vesicles using optically-induced dielectrophoresis on an integrated microfluidic platform," *Lab on a Chip,* vol. 21, no. 8, pp. 1475-1483, 2021.
[28] D. Zeng, N. Wu, L. Qian, H. Shi, and Y. Kang, "A novel controllable pneumatic needle-free injection system for larger-volume drug delivery," *Journal of Pharmaceutical Sciences,* vol. 109, no. 5, pp. 1772-1779, 2020.
[29] P. S. Chee, M. N. Minjal, P. L. Leow, and M. S. M. Ali, "Wireless powered thermo-pneumatic micropump using frequency-controlled heater," *Sensors and Actuators A: Physical,* vol. 233, pp. 1-8, 2015.
[30] T. Naito, "Development of microfluidic components for micro total analysis systems," *Chromatography,* 2020.
[31] C. Aracil, F. Perdigones, J. M. Moreno, A. Luque, and J. M. Quero, "Portable Lab-on-PCB platform for autonomous micromixing," *Microelectronic Engineering,* vol. 131, pp. 13-18, 2015.
[32] C. Huang and C. Tsou, "The implementation of a thermal bubble actuated microfluidic chip with microvalve, micropump and micromixer," *Sensors and actuators A: Physical,* vol. 210, pp. 147-156, 2014.
[33] A. Afzal and K.-Y. Kim, "Convergent–divergent micromixer coupled with pulsatile flow," *Sensors and Actuators B: Chemical,* vol. 211, pp. 198-205, 2015.
[34] M. Nafea, A. AbuZaiter, S. Kazi, and M. S. M. Ali, "Frequency-controlled wireless passive thermopneumatic micromixer," *Journal of Microelectromechanical Systems,* vol. 26, no. 3, pp. 691-703, 2017.
[35] J.-P. L. Bigué and J.-S. Plante, "Experimental study of dielectric elastomer actuator energy conversion efficiency," *IEEE/ASME Transactions on Mechatronics,* vol. 18, no. 1, pp. 169-177, 2011.
[36] F. A. M. Ghazali, C. K. Mah, A. AbuZaiter, P. S. Chee, and M. S. M. Ali, "Soft dielectric elastomer actuator micropump," *Sensors and Actuators A: Physical,* vol. 263, pp. 276-284, 2017.
[37] E. Acome *et al.*, "Hydraulically amplified self-healing electrostatic actuators with muscle-like performance," *Science,* vol. 359, no. 6371, pp. 61-65, 2018.
[38] Z. Suo, "Theory of dielectric elastomers," *Acta Mechanica Solida Sinica,* vol. 23, no. 6, pp. 549-578, 2010.

[39] M. R. Ahmad Fuaad, M. I. Ahmad Asri, and M. S. Mohamed Ali, "Self-healing Fluidic Dielectric Elastomer Actuator," in *Control, Instrumentation and Mechatronics: Theory and Practice*: Springer, 2022, pp. 252-260.

[40] T. Rehman, A.A. Mohd Faudzi, D.E.O. Dewi and M.S. Mohamed Ali, "Design, characterization, and manufacturing of circular bellows pneumatic soft actuator", *The International Journal of Advanced Manufacturing Technology*, vol. 93, pages 4295–4304, 2017.

[41] T. Rehman, M. Nafea, A.A. Mohd Faudzi, T. Saleh and M.S. Mohamed Ali, "PDMS-based dual-channel pneumatic micro-actuator", *Smart Materials and Structures*, vol. 28 (11), pages 115044, 2019.

CHAPTER 8

SMART TECHNOLOGIES FOR FATIGUE MONITORING THROUGH ARTIFICIAL INTELLIGENCE VIS-À-VIS IMPROVEMENT OF SAFETY IN THE MINING INDUSTRY

SINGAM JAYANTHU

Professor, Mining Engineering Department, National Institute of Technology, Rourkela - 769008, Odisha

ABSTRACT

This chapter discusses some of the technologies (artificial intelligence and machine learning) that are used to monitor and assess the fatigue levels of the personnel working in various capacities as vehicle drivers, conveyor operators, pump operators, or any moving machinery operators, etc., both in underground as well as surface mining conditions in the mining industry. Even if AI and ML algorithms can be of assistance in fatigue monitoring, the real reasons behind exhaustion can only be comprehended through research that employs technologies such as biomarkers. In recent years, it has become increasingly normal practice in the mining industry to use enormous fleets of machines with enormous capacities of shovels and dumpers. Despite the various technologies and methodologies, the human component plays an essential role in the operation and upkeep of the entire system, ensuring it is safe and effective. Because the majority of mining accidents result from carelessness on the part of the operator or heavy machinery, there is a pressing need to monitor the operator's level of productivity and awareness while working the machinery. The feeling of drowsiness or tiredness, as well as the associated physical and mental state of workers, is one of the primary contributors to accidents in the mining sector worldwide.

Keywords: *Health and Safety in Mining; Artificial Intelligence*

1. INTRODUCTION

The mining industry and other industries related to energy resources are associated with high rates of occupational injuries and deaths in most countries worldwide. This is especially true when compared to other industries. Mining is sometimes compared to waging war against the unpredictability of nature's elements. The mining industry continues to have a reputation for having a high rate of accidents, injuries, and illnesses as a direct consequence of this. Concerning the accidents that were caused by mining equipment, including dumpers and the need for fatigue monitoring requirements, this was reiterated in a recent Directorate General of Mines Safety (DGMS) Technical Circular # 6 of 2020, dated February 27, 2020, which outlined the basic design requirements and safety measures to be followed for heavy earth moving machinery and heavy/light vehicles in open cast mines for all coal and metalliferous mines [1].

Warning system for operator fatigue

An anti-sleepiness system that uses one or more ways to analyse operator fatigue symptoms allows the detection of drowsiness in the operator during the operation – driving. The technology promptly raises the alarm and visual alerts to notify the operator and others nearby. The reason why the system can do this is so it can analyse the many different symptoms that are related to operator weariness. The following is a list of the basic requirements and standards that the Warning System for Operator Fatigue needs to meet.

The computer should start up automatically at the same time as the engine or power supply of the machine, do an initial system check, and display an indicator that it is ready to use. The system will power down simultaneously with the engine or other source of power being turned off. To determine the system's condition, it must have an "ON" indicator, an initialisation indicator, a tracking indicator, and a signal that the system is malfunctioning. Essentially it detects drowsiness and generates an alarm to alert the operator and others in the vicinity to pay attention.

The system is to be comprised of the following four stages:

a) Initialisation: Each time the system is launched, it needs to be configured and optimised for the present user (Operator) and conditions. This process must be repeated each time the system is started. Therefore, the process of initialisation will be a relatively speedy one.

b) When discussing tracking, this means continuous surveillance of the person operating the machine inside a dynamically determined tracking region in real time.
c) Drowsiness Detection,
d) Warning: When it has been identified that the operator has been driving abnormally, the system will inform the driver of dangers that can develop as a result of this abnormal driving. A combination of auditory and visual warnings are used to draw the operator's attention and raise the level of attentiveness they are experiencing. An alerting system must be constructed in such a way as to prevent accidents from arising. For example, the system's components must not limit the range of motion, decrease the operator's field of view, or impede the machine's performance in any manner. In addition, it is required that the machine's components be made and installed in a way that prevents or minimises the effects of temperature, dust, dynamic loads, vibration, and shock that could cause the device to fail prematurely.

The system may be capable of recording the warning created along with a time stamp. This system will enable quick retrieval and analysis of the most recent 96 operational hours of deployment. Refer to DGMS Circulars and Indian and International Standards issued to determine the type, duration, and sound level of an audio warning and the intensity of an external visual warning.

The complicated state known as fatigue is defined by a lack of awareness and decreased mental and physical function, and it is frequently accompanied by drowsiness (1999 U.S. DOT Operational Definition). It is becoming more common knowledge that fatigue is a problem that affects the working population. Fatigue is a deadly outcome of a culture that functions 24 hours a day, according to research published by the National Safety Council, which finds that 13% of workplace injuries can be attributable to fatigue.

Most of the incidents are due to heavy earthmoving machinery, and the human element was the primary aspect contributing to the mishaps. Labour that is tedious and repetitive, as well as work that is performed around the clock, all contribute directly to increased levels of worker weariness. Several professions and sectors are plagued by a major ailment that can be summed up in one word: fatigue (World Health Organization, 1990). According to the Centers for Disease Control and Prevention in the United States (CDC, 2015), weariness is considered a public health hazard since one in every three persons does not obtain the recommended amount of sleep. Therefore, the safe completion of work must quantify and analyse the degrees of fatigue associated with each activity.

Two of the most important characteristics that need to be evaluated for each worker are their “severe weariness” and “limited functional capacity.” The symptoms of fatigue might present themselves in the body, the mind, or the emotions. The most important things to keep an eye out for to reduce the number of accidents that occur on the job are operator weariness and distraction. Common causes of weariness in mining environments include running machinery at night, inadequate illumination at the workplace, inadequate design of lighting systems, poor temperature settings at the workplace, noise, and excessively repetitive operations that result in boredom.

Smart Technologies for Fatigue Monitoring

The term “artificial intelligence” (AI) refers to the capacity of machines like computers and robots to perceive, reason, and carry out activities that people typically carry out. A subfield of artificial intelligence known as “machine learning” (ML) refers to algorithms designed to get smarter over time by being exposed to increasing data. Deep learning (DL) is one of the modern variants of machine learning techniques that allows the computer to think in a way the human thinks. It does this by learning from massive amounts of data.

Recommender engines are a product of machine learning. These engines suggest things that we might be interested in purchasing, movies that we might want to watch, or news articles that we might want to read. The development of natural language processing has made it feasible to translate between two languages in real-time, making it possible for two remote teams to communicate and increase overall productivity. Recent developments in deep learning have resulted in the creation of autonomous and self-driving automobiles, identifying a specific type of disease, and even dancing robots [2, 3].

Because of the hazardous nature of the work, the remote mine sites, and the high costs of personnel and transport, artificial intelligence (AI) and machine learning (ML) are two prime technologies that could benefit the mining industry. AI and ML have been used in various fields, including mineral prospecting, intelligent sorting of minerals and ores, demand forecasting, autonomous machinery, and many other areas. The applications of AI and ML in mining are still in their infancy, and more work requires to be done to achieve the full potential of these technological developments. Artificial intelligence has just recently begun to appear in the field of driver safety monitoring and fatigue management systems, particularly in the form of approaches involving computer vision and deep learning. Dotnetix.ai's Nexus, for example, monitors distracted driving situations with an in-cabin camera and sensor suite and sends data to a control centre. Visual analytics, an automated collision avoidance system, and body clock models are all utilised in hexagon mining.

As was discussed in the preceding sections, including fatigue, many different factors can contribute to weariness, including the following but not limited to work schedule, diet, sleep, personal habits, circadian cycles, long and repetitive work, exhaustion, medical causes, and psychological causes. To effectively monitor the operators and drivers for any signs of weariness, it is necessary to have a comprehensive picture of all of the factors that contribute to exhaustion. A holistic perspective, on the other hand, demands the ability to combine and comprehend information drawn from individuals' medical, social, behavioural, and physical records. To complete this operation manually is an exercise in futility. In addition, the data is often stored in silos and is almost certainly not in a format that can be automated. In addition, a real-time monitoring system is essential to provide the driver with timely warnings on issues and accidents [4–11].

Artificial intelligence has proven superior to human capabilities in several areas, particularly those that have reached their limits. The following is a list of some of the ways that AI can be used to monitor fatigue and ensure driver safety:

Technology 1: In-cabin camera to monitor the driver's physical state

The eyes may blink more slowly, the person may bob their head, their focus may wander, they may yawn, the steering wheel may move more slowly, there may be unexpected jerks in the adjustments, and so on. These are all physical indications of exhaustion. A camera that is oriented at the driver may determine, with the assistance of AI/ML, the key parameters indicative of the drowsiness by tracking eye movements, eyelid closure times, head movement, and hand movement during the operation. This allows the camera to determine whether the driver is attentive or is beginning to drift into an exhaustive condition. Studies have been performed for real-time eye blink detection by utilising facial landmarks, eye aspect ratio, and a support vector machine classifier to determine whether or not there was a blink. The ideas presented by Soukupova were pushed further by Baek et al., who then built an algorithm to identify tiredness in drivers. In addition, facial landmarks can be used to determine the direction that the head is facing. After the head movement has been tracked, a classifier algorithm is applied to determine whether the driver is exhibiting indicators of tiredness or distraction, such as staring at a cell phone for an extended period or looking to one side for an extended period. When combined with the historical data and the application of machine learning, the insights obtained by analysing the video data can be used to predict when the driver may begin to show signs of drowsiness, and corresponding corrective steps can be implemented at that time.

Technology 2: road monitoring system with optimal location predictor

The likelihood of identifying weariness and improving road safety can be increased by installing a camera facing forward on the road. The live feed from the camera is continuously watched to determine the route, as well as the ideal position in which the vehicle should be and its current location. Deep learning strategies, which are similar to the algorithms used in self-driving cars, are used to monitor the roads and determine the most effective position for the truck. The driver receives immediate and reliable input due to real-time processing at the edge (in the vehicle). The procedure is improved to monitor other machinery in the mining area, determine the distance between the truck and the other machines, and provide an early warning of any potential collisions with the other machines. Therefore, using this strategy provides the additional benefit of increased protection against the possibility of collisions. These kinds of strategies have, to the best of our knowledge, a significant amount of untapped potential but have not yet been used in the field.

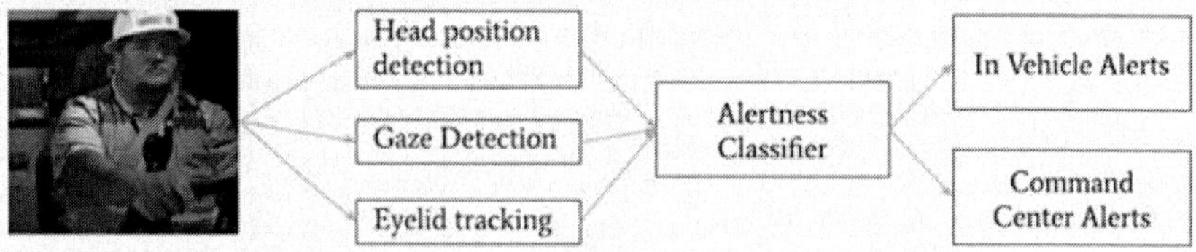

Figure 1: A typical driver safety monitoring system

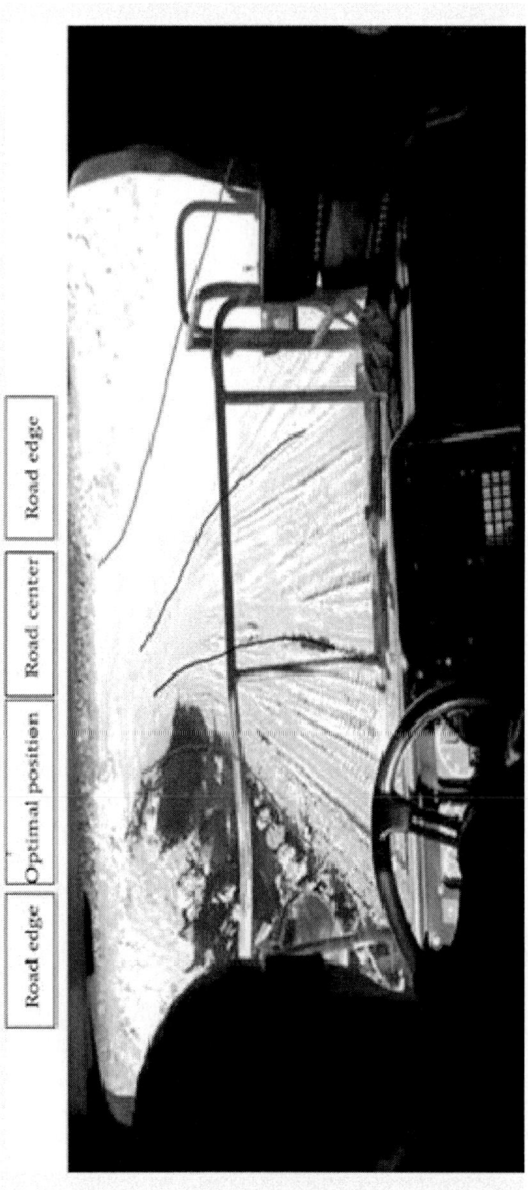

Figure 2. Road Monitoring Using Deep Learning

Technology 3: Ambient sensing technologies

It is well established that the surrounding environment can affect how a human body operates. For instance, Landstrom et al. [2] demonstrated that lowering the temperature within the cabin and keeping it there helps lessen the likelihood of drowsiness. Adding a sensor that can measure the surrounding temperature, humidity, and oxygen levels provides additional details. The data can be collected from the computer device or the sensors attached to the camera (edge nodes). In certain instances, the equipment might have sensors, the readings we can collect. When analysing the environmental data, one can gain insights that can be used to continuously alter the temperature inside the cabin to lessen the likelihood of being sleepy. In addition, the speed of the vehicle, its acceleration, the direction in which the steering wheel is turned, and other similar factors can be useful inputs for determining the driver's physical state. When combined with data from sensors located within the vehicle, data from sensors located outside the vehicle can be used to make more accurate predictions regarding the start of tiredness or distraction.

Technology 4: The driver's physical measurements

When a person is tired, physiological changes occur, including heart rate, blood pressure, and oxygen levels. The modifications begin when the body is just on the cusp of entering or emerging from a sleepy state. Monitoring these levels can provide us with more insights as well as early forecasts into the beginning stages of feeling sleepy. A health monitor band such as a Fitbit tracker can be used to monitor a person's heart rate, which can then determine whether or not the person is becoming drowsy. Having a tracker similar to Fitbit provides insight into a driver's physical activity during non-shift hours, which can be highly helpful in predicting potential problems that may arise due to a lack of sleep, exercise, or other activities. The user's heart rate, the amount of exercise they get, and how much they sleep are all things that many fitness trackers monitor. The ability to accurately forecast a person's physical state when they are operating machines may depend on information regarding their sleep activities. The task of monitoring multiple factors to anticipate drowsiness is a hard one. Combining data from a wide variety of sources and deriving insights from them has proven to be a very successful application of machine learning.

Technology 5: Combine the operator's medical records with the approaches above.

The physical and mental circumstances of an operator are extremely important factors in determining how susceptible they are to weariness. Therefore, it will be advantageous if medical records are combined to acquire further insights into future occurrences. Combining medical records, on the other hand, is not only technically difficult (due to a lack of standardisation of medical information) but also legally difficult (due to privacy laws such as HIIPA). As a result, the efficacy of this strategy in many regions of the world is questionable at best. However, in situations where it is feasible to do so, it is essential to include the patient's medical history to estimate the possibility of fatigue. Medical records form an important source of data which can be used to train deep learning models (AI/ML) to facilitate the assessment of the operators and the level of fatigue. It helps transform unstructured, free-form doctor's notes into structured data that can be further analysed using machine learning and has been used in several hospitals. These hospitals have used this power to gain insights into their patients' conditions.

Even if we showed the technologies that have the most benefits first and as additives to the ones that came before them, it is still possible to combine them in any sequence and acquire new perspectives. For instance, mining companies might decide to forego recording the driver to protect the driver's privacy and instead rely on the road monitoring system. In addition, a mining operation may want to simply evaluate how steering control occurs throughout the shift period to acquire insights about the state in which the driver is operating the vehicle.

Regardless of the strategy used, the data must be reviewed by the safety manager of the mining site, along with the operator(s) who were engaged in the occurrence. This must be done regardless of which approach is selected. Videos and the data collected from the sensors are saved for later examination and analysis to accomplish this goal. In addition, it is of the utmost importance to conduct mine-wide analyses of the accidents to keep track of where and when they occurred and who was involved in keeping the operations safe and improving the safety measures.

Biomarkers for Understanding Underlying Reasons

According to the official definition provided by the National Institutes of Health, a biomarker is "*a trait that is objectively tested and assessed as an indicator of normal pathogenic processes, biologic processes, or pharmacologic responses to a therapeutic intervention.*" This definition describes a biomarker as "*a trait that is objectively tested and assessed as an indicator of normal biologic processes, pathogenic processes, or pharmacologic responses*" (NIH). The Biomarkers Definitions Working Group published its findings in 2001. The concept of fatigue may be broken down into its parts, including the neurological, endocrine, and immune systems. Fatigue is a multifaceted construct of symptoms. The search for biomarkers that can diagnose chronic fatigue syndrome (CFS) is essential to this endeavour.

Further, it has been postulated that inflammation, activation of the immune system, dysfunction of the autonomic nervous system, reduced functioning of the hypothalamic-pituitary-adrenal axis, and dysregulation of neuroendocrine function are all primary causes of weariness. Even if AI and ML algorithms can assist fatigue monitoring, the real reasons behind exhaustion can only be comprehended through research that employs technologies such as biomarkers.

2. ACTION PLAN

Monitoring for fatigue is an essential step in ensuring that the mining operation continues to be safe, that its operators are protected, and that it continues to function efficiently. By implementing fatigue monitoring systems, mining operators can quickly begin to gain an advantage over their competitors. Gaussian Solutions LLC has worked with clients to create personalised solutions tailored to their needs. With the developments in mobile processing, it is possible to immediately start delivering mobile phone solutions. However, the viability of this strategy cannot be guaranteed. To achieve the reliability and availability required in the mining industry, specialised cameras and computing equipment at the edge of the network built to withstand the harsh conditions of the mines are necessary. In addition, for safety managers to monitor and take corrective actions, if a driver's lack of attentiveness is discovered, they need access to strong connectivity and real-time data.

Mining operators should approach the challenge with agility, and they should be able to rapidly deploy solutions, test them, and improve upon the deployments. A rapid development, deployment, test, monitor, and redo mantra should be implemented. To advance the overall state of safety measures in a mine, the mining community should have access to all of the evaluated data and the insights gathered. Finding an analytics and machine learning partner will help a mining firm progress faster and reach bigger results.

3. CONCLUSIONS

We are all susceptible to fatigue, notwithstanding our levels of talent, expertise, and understanding. Your physical and mental capabilities, which are required for even the simplest of tasks, are impacted. Because so many different things can cause or contribute to fatigue, there is no one certain technique to get rid of it. It is vital to take ideal measures in reducing fatigue, one that considers physical, emotional, situational, and environmental aspects. It is required to integrate the many systems that are currently available to monitor each of the factors. AI/ML is an effective way of processing data from various sources and deriving insights from them that can be used. Even if AI and ML algorithms can be of assistance in fatigue monitoring, the real reasons behind exhaustion can only be comprehended through research that employs technologies such as biomarkers.

It is possible that the operator, mining operations, and overall production could all benefit from the implementation of such techniques for fatigue monitoring. In the mining industry, there is an emphasis placed on the urgent implementation of transdisciplinary, industry-oriented research and academics, with some of the technologies (artificial intelligence and machine learning) used to monitor and assess the fatigue levels of the personnel working in various capacities as vehicle drivers, conveyor operators, pump operators, or any moving machinery operators, etc., both in underground as well as surface mining conditions. This is the case for mining operations in both underground and surface mining conditions. Increased operator productivity and a decrease in the number of incidents and accidents are both direct outcomes of fatigue monitoring's benefits.

REFERENCES

1. Minimum design requirements for various safety features to be incorporated in heavy earth moving machinery (HEMM) and heavy/light vehicles used in open cast mines, DGMS, 2020. DGMS (Tech) Circular No. O-6 of 2020, Dhanbad, dated 2/7/2020.
2. Landstorm, U.; Englund, K.; Nordstrom, B.; Stenudd, A. Use of Temperature Variations to Combat Drivers' Drowsiness. Percept. Mot. Skills 2002, 95, 497–506.

3. Tereza Soukupova and Jan' Cech, "Real-Time Eye Blink Detection Using Facial Landmarks," 21st Computer Vision Winter Workshop, February 2016.
4. J. W. Baek, B. Han, K. Kim, Y. Chung, and S. Lee, "Real-Time Drowsiness Detection Algorithm for Driver State Monitoring Systems," 2018 Tenth International Conference on Ubiquitous and Future Networks (ICUFN), Prague, 2018, pp. 73–75, DoI: 10.1109/ICUFN.2018.8436988.
5. Who is at Risk for Fatigue? National Safety Council https://www.nsc.org/workplace/safety-topics/fatigue/fatigue-whos-at-risk?
6. Convert Your Resource Into Value, Tomra, https://www.tomra.com/en/sorting/mining

CHAPTER 9

HOW AI/ML/DL IS ASSISTING IN THE EFFECTIVE REHABILITATION OF LOWER LIMB AMPUTEES?

RAVI KANT AVVARI

Department of Biotechnology and Medical Engineering, National Institute of Technology Rourkela, Odisha – 769 008, India

ABSTRACT

Amputation is the removal of the part of the body giving an unforeseen injury or infection, such as trauma (accidents, occupational hazards), tumour formation, frostbite and non-traumatic events via surgical means. With an increasing incidence of lower-limb amputation (23,500 amputees/year in India comprising 20,200 males and 3,300 females), there is a considerable demand for an active prosthesis to serve the function of the lost part of the limb. Besides having a prosthesis, there is also a need for rehabilitation to gain muscle strength post-surgery through exercising and improving the range of mobility towards normal. Whereas passive devices provide locomotion with limited mobility with some flexibility, and active prosthesis requires the intelligence to determine the user's intention to move, developing a hybrid prosthesis with advantages of passive and active ones is an increasing challenge. Artificial intelligence has been instrumental in designing prostheses that would achieve specifications of efficient design involving less energy during exertion and better ambulation with less involvement. This chapter introduces the state of the art in creating prostheses using AI/ML for effective rehabilitation.

Keywords: *Lower limb amputees; Artificial intelligence; Machine learning; Deep learning; Kalman filter; Rehabilitation*

1. INTRODUCTION

Amputation is the removal of the part of the body giving an unforeseen injury or infection, such as trauma (accidents, occupational hazards), tumour formation, frostbite and non-traumatic events via surgical means. The series of events, post-injury, leads to further damage to the tissue if proper precautions are not taken. In non-traumatic circumstances, a typical situation is poor blood circulation in the affected regions due to the narrowing of blood vessels, as in limbs, which reduces the supply of oxygenated blood to the tissues, leading to ischemia (peripheral artery disease). In severity, and in cases where the possible restoration of blood supply is not feasible, it may lead to critical limb ischemia. In the diabetic foot, not so uncommon can lead to complications from nerve injury to the onset of peripheral artery disease and infection. Due to a lack of oxygen and nutrients, the tissue becomes more susceptible to further damage and infection, causing gangrene (gas, dry and wet forms). The gangrene, if it starts emerging and is potentially harmful to the tissues surrounding it. As it may spread quickly to neighbouring tissues, immediate medical attention is required.

Lower limb amputation (LLA) is a last resort of surgery to save the patient from losing another limb section due to further damage caused by the quick spreading of the infection (due to saprogenic microorganisms). LLA challenges the existence of the living psychologically and physically. It limits physical accessibility, increases the burden of doing the task and reduces the quality of life. Unfortunately, the problem is common and remains invisible. Besides the lower-limb amputation (23,500 amputees/year in India comprising 20,200 males and 3,300 females), a considerable number of 5,436,000 Indians also suffer from locomotor disability (Census 2011, India).

Post amputation, patients are allowed for rehabilitation involving regaining mobility through a prosthesis. During the pre-prosthesis phase, they undergo sessions/therapy to prepare the limb for a prosthesis, such as building muscle strength. This is followed by the prosthetic preparation for the amputee based on the prosthesis's shape, size requirement, and utility. Finally, training sessions are followed to gain control of the device during locomotion. In this context, the level of rehabilitation intervention required is individual-specific. Through rehabilitation, we intend to assess the improvement in the locomotion with prosthesis and how best the patient can control and regain functionality; if possible, we devise rehabilitation strategies to improve.

In this chapter, the concept of rehabilitation is introduced for lower limb amputees, discussing the state-of-the-art strategies available for regaining mobility as best as possible. Furthermore, since locomotion is highly variable and individual-centric, movement sensing is mandated to ensure proper control of the prosthesis actuated by the onboard motors as additional support. Here we also discuss how the sensor fusion technologies help realise the prosthesis, which could make the patients feel the artificial limb via feedback sensing. Finally, concerning the previous success stories of rehabilitation using a bionic limb, we discuss state-of-the-art bionic limb design using AI/ML/DL techniques, followed by future design directions.

2. REHABILITATION STRATEGIES FOR LOWER LIMB AMPUTEES

Post-surgical trauma of amputation can be a disturbing phase leading to post-traumatic stress disorder. By losing the limb, there is a loss of an essential part of the limb involved in the movement. As a result, there is a loss of sensation and functionality. Depending on the type of lower limb amputation, the sensation and functionalities are affected accordingly. Typical amputation includes – hemipelvectomy, hip disarticulation, very short above knee, above the short knee, medium above the knee, long above the knee, knee disarticulation, short below the knee, standard below the knee in lower limb; amputation (Syme's, Chopart, Lisfranc, transmetatarsal, and toe), and Metatarsophalangeal disarticulation in the foot.

To adapt to continual challenges, clinicians refer to rehabilitation centres for possible adaption. Because there is a loss of the limb, there is a need for the recovery or gain of the function that is lost due to LLA. Living with the physical limitation to move around and perform routine tasks is challenging.

Rehabilitation provides opportunities for regaining the lost functionalities. By rehabilitation, we refer to preparation and adaption to do physically challenging tasks with the help of prosthetics/ bionics. During the preparatory phase, the subjects are administered a series of exercises to improve muscle strength and control. If required, prosthetics/ bionics can facilitate balancing the body to assist in locomotion. Rehabilitation is a discipline of relevance to interdisciplinary engineering that promotes and regains lost functionalities. It helps to develop technologies to recover the functions through the use of supports, either independently or partially, to carry out daily activities in their life. This not only serves to gain partial/ full functionality but also provides emotional support in the sense of a limb being artificial.

In brief, the rehabilitation for the lower limb amputee involves strategies such as,

- functional training to improve muscle strength post-surgery
    - for example, exercising for isometric contractions at the peak of the isotonic movement will be useful for gaining strength
    - gaining sufficient trunk strength to cope with mobility and avoiding gait deviations
- functional assessment of the significant muscle groups contributing to good force generation for reliable movement
- evaluation of the kinematic features for the residual limb's range of motion
- evaluation of the extent of immobility for the possible design of the prosthesis
- use of tools/ devices to assist in strengthening the residual limb for isotonic and isokinetic strengthening

As discussed in the following sections, further advancements in rehabilitation are proving a success in prosthetic designs from being artificial to a close representation of the lost limb in the sense of having an innate biofeedback response.

3. STATE OF THE ART IN REHABILITATION ENGINEERING

The purpose of rehabilitation is to develop an artificial substitute for the lost part of the body that could integrate with the human body to serve the purpose of the lost functionality and be a close representation of the lost part (Fishman, 1977). For example, lower limb prosthesis has advanced remarkably in the recent past with an intent to devise a bionic substitute of the part of the limb to regain the loss of function in terms of kinematics and kinetics.

Commercially available devices can be classified as passive, active and semi-active prostheses. Passive ones are designed to have a non-flexible actuation using a hydraulic (**GENIUM**) actuator adjusted to have the desired amount of damping into the system to sustain a sufficient amount of the rotational forces during the knee flexion (maximum 130°); designed to obtain the best response for protection from fall. Passive devices rely on the force due to the body movement to cause the motion. While in active ones, the forces are provided using actuators such as motors to process the force to cause the motion. Active devices (**EmPOWER**) help restore mobility with little assistance from the subject. It, however, weighs heavier than the passive ones, as it comes with onboard actuators and supports (gear system and mechanical accessories).

Nonetheless, the design provides mechanical support to facilitate the movement in partial/ complete loss of function of the limb motion. These devices assist in performing routine tasks, such as the normal movement of the limbs, in achieving a partial or complete gain of locomotion. This requires ensuring the design has a symmetrical distribution of weight about the central axis and balancing ability during locomotion, allowing for a typical gait pattern. Improvisation of the device is always possible, with design specifications meeting the gait patterns as close to the healthy individuals. This requires testing the devices, training sessions to adapt the device and post-training assessment to validate the rehabilitation during the rehabilitation.

In prosthesis involving ankle rehabilitation, motorising the ankle flexion allows for better movement for negligible or no-load-bearing tasks, typically during the swing phase. Such a real-time motion requires fusion of the prosthesis with the sensor (sensor fusion) involving sensors such as an inertial sensor (accelerometer, gyroscope), strain gauges, and goniometer, which allows for estimating measuring anterior and posterior bending moment. Precise estimation of the joint angle during gait phases is necessary to introduce necessary actuation during the stance and swing phases. Whereas not all the phases of the gait cycle are replicable, part of the dynamics can be mimicked using – 1) powered knee prostheses for recreation of early-stance knee flexion and extension and 2) powered ankle prostheses for the addition of additional energy for powered push-off. Active prostheses improve the quality of the gait prosthesis, especially by driving the traction system to recreate the gait pattern as observable during a regular walk. In addition, it enhances the functionalities of the prosthesis with freedom for correcting the gait cycle through the motorising prosthesis. However, motorisation increases the weight of the prosthesis and the inertia contributing to increased power requirement, which is a disadvantage. In such cases, both passive and active elements are used for an optimal design for the (hybrid) prostheses. Such design usually employs elastic actuators in various configurations, serial, parallel, or a combination, to achieve the desired mechanical response (Rouse, 2014).

The bionic limb employs the actuation of the traction system via feedback sensing. Feedback sensing involves using implantable devices for neuro sensing done via a surgical procedure, as in devices with neural implants. These neural implants help in recording the neurons' activity at the target muscles' levels through direct interfacing with neurons. Such prosthesis involving the implantation of the chip costs more and is not affordable to many, despite many disadvantages as to infection and reduced acceptability by the patient. Biofeedback in sensing using inertial sensors is a promising solution for low-cost and affordable bionic limbs. Wearable sensors employing inertial sensors such as accelerometers and gyros have been well studied in the literature in diverse environments (indoor, outdoor, rough terrain). Cockcroft et al. show the potential use of the wireless sensor in estimating dynamic acceleration and calculating hip angles during cycling (J. Cockcroft, 2014). Hand and Foot trajectory of sports persons playing cycling (J. Cockcroft, 2014; James Y. Xu, 2015) to golf (Y. J. Kim, 2017), table tennis (X. Sha, 2021) to gymnastics (V. Bonnet, 2013) can be observed using these sensors. Cockcroft et al. show the potential use of the wireless sensor in estimating dynamic acceleration and calculating hip angles during cycling (J. Cockcroft, 2014). Hand and foot trajectory of sports persons playing cycling (J. Cockcroft, 2014; James Y. Xu, 2015) to golf (Y. J. Kim, 2017), table tennis (X. Sha, 2021) to gymnastics (V. Bonnet, 2013) can be determined using these sensors. While these sensors suffer from drift errors, deep learning strategies have been employed to further enhance the quality of risk assessment, such as SVM, KNN, NB, RF, MLP, and CNN, with reasonable accuracy, sensitivity and specificity (Howcroft, 2016; Qiu, 2018; Wang, 2020). Recent studies on using pressure sensors with inertial sensors with a novel multisource CNN ensemble framework reported promising results in pre-impact fall detection (Wang, 2020).

In assistive rehabilitation, where the possibility of cure and rehabilitation is a subject of debate, possibilities of betterment and improved quality of life, as assessed from the questionnaire with bionic limbs, cannot be ignored. Bionic limbs offer a better rehabilitation platform than traditional task-specific repetitive training (treadmill training and passive prosthesis). However, the theoretical rationale of the rehabilitation is not convincing or may require better modalities for assessing the change in gait pre/post rehabilitation. Furthermore, there is insufficient understanding as far as the evidence is concerned to establish the biomechanics of rehabilitation in terms of the control variables.

The bionic limb can facilitate targeted neural rehabilitation to regain the functions of neural sensing and actuation. Furthermore, studies aim to exploit neural plasticity, considering the hypothesis that central nervous system (CNS) and peripheral nervous system (PNS) circuits adapt to motor learning activities, enabling flexibility in reorganising its structure, functions, and connections.

4. DESIGN OF BIONIC LIMB FOR AMPUTEES

Depending upon the loss of locomotion function, the prosthesis is designed to gain the function as much as possible. Passive devices (as in transtibial prosthesis) are driven by force due to the movement of the affected limb; there is no substantial improvement in locomotion. Such prostheses do not allow for necessary kinematic and kinetic adjustments and constraints locomotion with limited mobility in the workspace accessible. Therefore, the prosthesis should be designed to have a certain flexibility and sufficient degrees of freedom to ensure a close approximation to the normal gait pattern of a healthy individual. Bionics is the preferred choice of the prosthesis as it allows for active traction of the motorised prosthesis for executing the gait pattern in synchronism with the other limb. Literature studies indicate that combined passive and active prostheses (or hybrid) show promising results in efficient design involving less energy during exertion, ambulating more efficiently up stairs and ramps, and performing sit-to-stand transitions more easily. Likewise, numerous challenges are present, requiring improvisation of the technical design following hybrid or combined passive and active design approaches. The objective of the hybrid prosthesis is to mimic the natural movement of the lost limbs by integrating the biological aspects of sensing (feedback sensing) with the prosthesis in a well-coordinated manner to perform the traction.

A more affordable solution would be improvising the current design through sensor fusion technology with the prosthesis. The use of inertial sensors (accelerometer, gyro) with deep learning strategies can be a potential modality to supplement the neuro sensing for the bionic limb. Recent studies indicate better precision in estimating the gait, which can be fed back to the onboard computer for generating the neural signal for actuating the traction unit. Surface EMG markers also assist in estimating neural signals developed by the amputated part of the limb in the feedback sensing and actuation control. Growing knowledge of the use of MEMS-based sensor and EMG markers in gait show great potential in exploring design without implanting any electrodes, a great relaxation for the patients. Further, the technology also facilities rehabilitation (improved gait speed, step length, ankle power) in locomotive syndrome patients. Such ideas will improve muscle strength, balance, and gait symmetry with less dependency on the prosthesis.

5. SENSOR FUSION TECHNOLOGIES – FEEDBACK SENSING

To develop the prosthesis for the lower extremities, sufficient information on the gait pattern of the subject is essential. With disability, normal gait patterns are lost, and with amputation, the control aspects of balancing are disturbed completely. Therefore, the prosthesis needs to have the intelligence to control the actuation of the motors to drive the motion of the artificial limb in synchronous with the user's intention. In this section, we describe how gait analysis plays an essential role in understanding the gait pattern of the subjects and how this information can be integrated to develop such intelligence to actuate the active prosthesis to work in synchronism with the user's intention for lower limb movement.

Sensor fusion is a technology whereby, using many sensors, we establish the intelligence to assess the sensor data and determine the control action to drive the actuators (traction system of the active prosthesis) by intentions.

Inertial sensors such as accelerometers, gyroscopes, goniometers and magnetometers are used to detect the movement of the limb. Several such sensors are placed on the limb and torso to study the gait. Most commonly, the accelerometers as single sensors or in combination with a gyroscope are used to study the limb movement, finally deducing the kinematics of the motion. As these sensors are tiny, it is embedded and used as part of the wearable to enhance the study. In addition, information about the time history of the changes in the acceleration of the specific location on the limb is studied. The sensor is generally worn over the hand or legs to facilitate wireless measurement and recording. Several sensors are placed over the limb to study the movement of various locations about the joint position and reference coordination in the local frame of reference. Further, with many sensors, artefacts arising from sensor-related movements/ placement issues can be readily suppressed or eliminated to a greater extent. Since this is easy to wear and study the gait, the technology has been widely researched to detect the gait phases during the online measurement and determine the user's intention or the transition in locomotion modes.

Additional sensors, such as plantar sensors, are also used to capture the pressure field left behind during foot and ground contact. This information is useful to correlate with inertial data and deduce the step-by-step movement as a collaborative effort to detect the gait phases precisely. Sensors employing EMG (electromyography) markers are also used to detect limb-specific information as to the grasp force, feedback-driven corrections, and latency in the user grip to improve proprioceptive sensing.

EMG sensors can adaptively predict the active kinetic details of the lower limb, provide calibration, and an efficient algorithm is used to remove the artefacts and noise. EMG in gait analysis can be beneficial to predict the sub-phases of the gait and events at the level of the skeletal muscle system of the lower limb. Details of the onset of contraction of the muscles (to name a few - Tibialis Anterior, Lateral Gastrocnemius, and Rectus Femoris) can be corrected with the gait phases to enhance our understanding of the user's intention and development of algorithms for prediction of the next transition in locomotion modes.

The motivation for feedback sensing has been to reconstruct the lost functionalities of motor control of the lower limb in association with the central nervous system. With gait measures, we also tend to know the change in the gait pattern during rehabilitation, pre/post-surgical interventions and training sessions. From a clinical point of view, the study of electrical potential may provide further information on rehabilitation that may not be possible from inertial sensing (Agostini V., 2020). Though EMG provides direct access to the muscular function, there is a certain amount of ambiguity and challenges, which include a lack of normative data on electromyogram, repeatability, reproducibility and lack of clinical markers to distinguish precisely the events during rehabilitation.

Researchers have been trying to establish the lost proprioception sensing artificially in a very ambitious effort. In amputation, there is a loss of sensation and motor control. As a result, the sensory and motor nerves are removed, partially or wholly, to render the limb inactive to case motion even with the prosthesis. On-going efforts to re-establish the sensory-motor systems show signs of futuristic designs that may help recover the lost mobility and sensing abilities of the limb. The state of art research involves connecting an amputee's residual musculature and the functional nervous tissue. With newer technologies such as targeted muscle reinnervation (TMR) and targeted sensory reinnervation (TSR), establishing the bidirectional communication between the brain and the peripheral system (PNS and Limb muscles) is possible (Marasco, P. D., 2021).

6. ROLE OF AI/ML/DL IN REHABILITATION ENGINEERING

AI has emerged as one of the most successful technologies as it imitates human-like abilities in decision-making and prediction. It is these capabilities which, based on the factual information and the previous information and training, AI tools have been able to predict future events as best as possible reliably. Even if the tool may not predict the next event, after further training, it improvises its learning patterns to assess future events as close as possible to reality.

To track the movement accurately, we prefer using an inertial sensor to measure the acceleration data and integrate it twice to determine the position information. Having the accelerometer sensor allows measurement of the acceleration of the particular location; similarly, having the gyroscope allows measurement of the angle-pitch and roll angles. The gyroscope measures angular velocity in deg/s which, upon integration, gives the angle in degrees. However, such direct integration of the sensor data does not give rise to accurate measurement owing to drift errors. It would be readily observed that after a few seconds, the position information is already drifted by some units away from actuals.

Furthermore, we notice a drift in the quantity measurement, which also increases over time. In addition, with integration, these errors are summed up to give erroneous linear and rotational positions. Thus, it shows that we need more than merely sensor data analysis for reliable results. Hence, algorithms are to be designed to overcome the issues of drift errors.

Tracking algorithms such as the Kalman filter have been trendy when tracking a moving object (Basu P., 2022). Further, with a single sensor, there are issues relating to the noise, which also limits the tracking accuracy. Therefore, one of the solutions is to use two sensors to eliminate/ suppress the errors, as discussed in the following.

Consider an example of two sensors placed at the end of the shank. As we know, the accelerometer measures the acceleration components along the three perpendicular directions. According to Newton's law of motion, accelerations can be represented mathematically for the system with two sensors as follows:

$$\mathbf{a}_2 = \frac{d^2\mathbf{r}_2}{dt^2} - \mathbf{g} = \ddot{\mathbf{r}}_0 + \frac{\ddot{\mathbf{l}}}{2} - \mathbf{g} \qquad \mathbf{a}_1 = \frac{d^2\mathbf{r}_1}{dt^2} - \mathbf{g} = \ddot{\mathbf{r}}_0 - \frac{\ddot{\mathbf{l}}}{2} - \mathbf{g}$$

[1]

Where r_0 is the position vector of the centre of the rod, and g is the acceleration due to gravity. Taking the difference of the acceleration from these two sensors, the vector I can be derived independent of the gravitational effects,

$$\ddot{\mathbf{l}} = l\ddot{\phi}\mathbf{u}_0 - l\dot{\phi}^2\mathbf{l}_0 = l\alpha\mathbf{i}_x - l\omega^2\mathbf{i}_y, \quad [2]$$

where φ is the angle between the axes x (perpendicular to the vector l) and x', ω and α are the rod's absolute angular velocity and angular acceleration, respectively.

The difference in the acceleration in the direction along the rod axis depends on the square of the angular velocity and the angular acceleration. The two sensors eliminated the problem of gravity components and noise resulting from the signal. Now that the issues of noise were minimised using the two-sensor system, we can focus on the estimation of the joint angles and reduction of the drift with the help of digital filtering. The angular acceleration of the knee can be smoothened further using a low pass and high pass filter. The choice of cut-off frequency, f_0, is done through heuristic means to assess the drift reduction. Although the use of filtering by choice of f_0 reduces the drift, it does not allow generalising the algorithm. Therefore, it requires further analysis of how one could extract drift in terms of filtering. While this could be a potential solution to the drift problem, we also sought drift estimation and elimination by using other methods, such as Kalman filtering.

The Kalman filter, also known as linear quadratic estimation (LQE), is used to model linear systems to predict the state space by achieving a minimum variance estimate of the state through iteration. They are also used for real-time applications, basically for online estimation of the state variable based on the knowledge of the prior state of the system or process. The advantage of the Kalman filter is the ability to predict the best estimate of the next state closely, given – noisy sensor data and uncertainty in the process.

A formal solution to the above problem is shown for an Extended Kalman Filter (EKF),

$$\textbf{Initialisation :}\quad \mathbf{X_0} = E[X_t]$$

$$\mathbf{P_0} = E[(X_0 - X_t)(X_0 - X_t)^T]$$

$$\textbf{Predict step :}\quad X_{k|k-1} = f(X_{k-1|k-1}, u_{k-1})$$

$$P_{k|k-1} = F_{k-1}P_{k-1|k-1}F_{k-1}^T + \mathbf{Q}$$

$$\textbf{Update step :}\quad K_k = P_{k|k-1}H_k^T(H_kP_{k|k-1}H_k^T + \mathbf{R})^{-1}$$

$$X_{k|k} = X_{k|k-1} + K_k(Z_k - h(X_{k|k-1}))$$

$$P_{k|k} = (I - K_kH_k)P_{k|k-1}$$

[3]

where the variables are defined as follows,

True initial state $:X_t$

Initial state estimate $:X_{0|0} = \mathbf{X_0}$

Initial state covariance matrix $:P_{0|0} = \mathbf{P_0}$

State Jacobian matrix $:F_{k-1} = \left[\frac{\partial f}{\partial X}\right]_{X=X_{k-1|k-1}}$

Measurement Jacobian matrix $:H_k = \left[\frac{\partial h}{\partial X}\right]_{X=X_{k|k-1}}$

[4]

For drift reduction, the choice of cut-off frequency, f_0, can be made through heuristic means to assess the drift reduction. However, although the use of filtering by choice of f_0 reduces the drift, it does not allow generalising the algorithm. Therefore, it requires further analysis of how one could extract drift in terms of filtering. While this could be a potential solution to the drift problem, we also sought drift estimation and elimination by using other methods, such as Kalman filtering. The Kalman filter, also known as linear quadratic estimation (LQE), is used to model linear systems to predict the state space by achieving a minimum variance estimate of the state through iteration.

Although the use of filtering by choice of f_0 reduces the drift, it does not allow generalising the algorithm. Therefore, it requires further analysis of how one could extract drift in terms of filtering. While this could be a potential solution to the drift problem, we also sought drift estimation and elimination by using other methods, such as Kalman filtering.

The study will also explore extended KF and cascaded KF, ZUPT and other algorithms for improved estimation of the gait. ZUPT has particular relevance to the project. MEMS-based IMU sensors are extensively used for estimating the trajectory of the foot. However, the large amount of drift present in the sensors should be removed beforehand. Zero-velocity update method (ZUPT) helps in minimising the drift in IMU sensors. During a fraction of the time in the midstance, the velocity and acceleration of the heel are precisely zero. Without this correction, the sensor drift increased for a few meters in four to five steps. The stance phase detection is almost a pattern recognition process, where the stance phase is observed under two circumstances – acceleration should be close to g since the x- and y-axis of a calibrated accelerometer is 0, and that of the z-axis is close to 9.81. Angular velocity will be 0 since, for a calibrated gyroscope, all the axis are 0. The single detection threshold method is the conventional stance detection method of the ZUPT algorithm. This method compares the IMU acceleration and angular velocities with the ZUPT acceleration threshold and ZUPT angular velocity threshold, respectively.

Based on the described joint angle estimation algorithm, we sought to calibrate the measurement by comparing it with the measurement obtained using a camera capture system. As mentioned in the algorithm, we use the two sensors system mounted on a rigid rod to estimate the joint angle. To reduce the drift or errors in the measurement during the run, we seek for estimation of the drift and elimination from the measurement by utilising the Kalman filter. The final joint angle estimate by an enhanced version of the KF will be compared with those obtained by the camera capture system and goniometer. Numerous measurements will be taken and assessed for confidence in estimating the joint angle for various movements with the help of a statistical tool (SPSS).

As is evident from the literature, numerous motion-tracking algorithms have been investigated to explore the most reliable one for the study of gait. However, such algorithms become very much biased to the study and experiment setup context.

Deep learning provides amazing opportunities to scope better algorithms in motion sensing with sensor fusion. DL offers an intuitive way of mimicking the human-like brain to automatically detect the features that could help detect the pattern and differentiate the data based on these features selected by the neural network architecture trained to do so. The three fundamental network architectures utilised to achieve such intelligence that is based on the following - Convolutional Neural Networks (CNN), Recurrent Neural Networks (RNN), and Recursive Neural Networks. In contrast to ML, deep learning algorithms analyse the dataset thoroughly and learn to identify/distinguish features that may be useful in delineating the subject into different groups. For example, in CNN, the images are convoluted at various levels to perform feature analysis through various stages. This way, it intuitively recognises the distinct features which can form the basis of separating the data into distinct groups. AI/ML/DL has been widely employed in the sensor data (inertial sensor, EEG) to determine best the gait phases for possible actuation of the active prosthesis. However, the challenge is how well it distinguishes the user's motion intent and transition in the locomotion modes. Table 1 shows various rehabilitation studies of lower limb amputees using artificial intelligence in the context of lower limb prosthesis, where AI/ML/DL techniques have been used for reliable design prototyping with increased accuracy; the past three years of literature data.

7. SUMMARY

Prosthesis design has been a challenge, especially for lower limb amputees, where the active prosthesis needs to be controlled in line with the user's intention. For a good design, there needs to be scope for better sensing which forms the proprioceptive part of the bionic limb. Since machine learning strategies are move-biased, researchers have been shifting towards deep learning strategies to improve the reliability of gait measurement - gait phases and user's intention, including the transition of the locomotion modes. Improvements in existing deep learning methods and better proprioceptive feedback sensing design are state-of-art in the area. This not only allows for better actuation of the prosthesis but also allows for monitoring the improvement in patient locomotion and rehabilitation.

Table 1: Rehabilitation studies of lower limb amputees using artificial intelligence – AI/ ML/ DL – studies from past three years till Jan 2023

Author	Investigation	Subject	Activity or Dataset, if any	Outcome measures	Methods	Observations
Juneau P. et al., 2022	fall risk classification	80 nos. (27 fallers, 53 non-fallers)	6-minute walk test (6MWT) using a smartphone	Step features – temporal, statistical and frequency	LSTM	Foot strikes were correctly identified in 58 of 80 participants with an accuracy of 72.5%; provide opportunities for the mobile app for fall risk assessment
Griffiths B. et al., 2021	To identify postures (sitting, standing, stepping, and lying)	12 males, three females	Observation of daily activity	3-axis acceleration data	Random Forest Classifier	Machine learning classification model can be used to identify postures with an accuracy of 93%,
Pergolini A. et al., 2022	improve walking using a powered hip exoskeleton	Four transfemoral amputees	Sit-to-stand/stand-to-sit and dynamic motion	Hip angles, foot longitudinal axis CoP	Real-Time LRA using LDA classifier	Further experimentations of the technology essential to improve the technique for LLA
Murray R. et al., 2022	Struggles with mobility	Seven subjects with a transfemoral amputation	Locomotion modes - sitting, standing, level-ground walking, and motion involving ramps and stairs.	Kinematic and sonography data	Combined sonography and kinematic network	There is higher reliability for assessing transitions between ambulation modes with opportunities to overcome challenges of walking over different terrains

Daines K. J., 2021	Fall-risk assessment	89 amputees	6-minute walk test using a smartphone	Accelerometer and gyroscope data	Correlation-based feature selection, random forest classifier	The study reduced the time of assessing the risk factors associated with falls and was useful in clinical evaluation while reducing patient time in clinics
Khan A. T., 2023	Role of the central nervous system in vibrotactile feedback in EEG	Three transfemoral amputees	Weight-shifting exercises	EEG data	kNN classifier	Spinocerebellum and Cerebro-cerebellum are useful in directional motor planning and control.
Liang F. Y., (2022).	Role of the nervous system in muscle synergies	Eight unilateral transfemoral amputee	Walk at their self-selected speeds	Acceleration, angular velocity, and quaternion	CRP, PCA, LSTM	LSTM offers a better assessment of the synergy, which is very useful in prosthesis design
Stolyarov R., (2020).	Develop terrain prediction algorithms.	Five below-knee amputations	Walking trials - level ground, stairs, and ramps	Sensor data	Heuristic back-estimation	Able to predict at less than 2.8% error on all strides
Su B. Y., 2019	Predict motion intent in amputees	One transtibial amputee	Locomotion mode (level ground, stairs, and ramp)	Inertial sensors	Convolutional neural network	Obtained an accuracy of 89.23% for amputees on user's motion intent

Marcos Mazon D., 2022	Detect transitions and gait phases	One osseointegrated transfemoral amputee subject	Sitting, standing, level ground walking, ramp and stair movement.	ENABL3S data set, MyLeg data set -	Multi-level architecture - CNN, CNN-GRU, or CNN-LSTM	CNN-LSTM networks can correctly classify with a mean F1-score of 0.89/0.92
Karakish M., 2022	Tracking of lower limb motion for active prosthesis control	Unilateral amputee (for study on active prophesies)	Walking, running, and stairs movement	HuGaDB Dataset, inertial sensors (accelerometer and gyroscope)	Deep Multi-Layer Perceptron, Deep CNN	CNN can reliably predict lower limbs kinematics in comparison to MLP
de Mendonça Mesquita E., 2020	Classification of Lower limb amputee groups	Transtibial and transfemoral amputees	Treadmill walking - horizontal, up and down the hill	Gait data	KNN, RF	A classification accuracy of 75.8% and 77.7% for KNN and RF was obtained

* Electroencephalography (EEG); Short-Term Long Memory (LSTM); Linear Discriminant Analysis (LDA); Locomotion Recognition Algorithm (LRA); Center of Pressure (CoP); Continuous Relative Phase (CRP); Principal Component Analysis (PCA); HuGaDB (Human Gait Database); K-nearest neighbours (KNN); random forest (RF); Encyclopedia of Able-bodied Bilateral Lower Limb Locomotor Signals (ENABL3S); study also involved healthy subjects where possible in facilitating the data analysis with able-bodied.

REFERENCES

1. Basu, P., & Avvari, R. K., Prospects of Wearable Inertial Sensors for Assessing Performance of Athletes Using Machine Learning Algorithms. In Image Processing and Intelligent Computing Systems (pp. 137–151). CRC Press.
2. Howcroft J, Lemaire ED, Kofman J. Wearable-sensor-based classification models of faller status in older adults. PLoS One. 2016;11(4):e0153240.
3. Wang, L., Peng, M., and Zhou, Q. (2020). Pre-impact fall detection based on multisource CNN ensemble. IEEE Sensors J. 20, 5442–5451. doi: 10.1109/JSEN.2020.2970452
4. Qiu, (2018). Application of Wearable Inertial Sensors and A New Test Battery for Distinguishing Retrospective Fallers from Non-fallers among Community-dwelling Older People.
5. V. Bonnet, C. Mazza, P. Fraisse, A. Cappozzo, "Real-time Estimate of Body Kinematics During a Planar Squat Task Using a Single Inertial Measurement Unit", IEEE TRANSACTIONS ON BIOMEDICAL ENGINEERING, VOL. 60, NO. 7, JULY 2013, Page: 1920-1926.
6. James Y. Xu et al., "Integrated Inertial Sensors and Mobile Computing for Real-Time Cycling Performance Guidance via Pedalling Profile Classification", IEEE JOURNAL OF BIOMEDICAL AND HEALTH INFORMATICS, VOL. 19, NO. 2, MARCH 2015, Page No.: 440–445.
7. Y. J. Kim et al., "Golf Swing Analysis System with a Dual Band and Motion Analysis Algorithm", IEEE Transactions on Consumer Electronics, Vol. 63, No. 3, August 2017, Page No.: 309–317.
8. X. Sha et al., "Accurate Recognition of Player Identity and Stroke Performance in Table Tennis Using a Smart Wristband", IEEE SENSORS JOURNAL, VOL. 21, NO. 9, MAY 1, 2021, Page No.: 10923–10932.
9. J. Cockcroft, J.H. Muller, C. Scheffer, "A Novel Complimentary Filter for Tracking Hip Angles During Cycling Using Wireless Inertial Sensors and Dynamic Acceleration Estimation", IEEE SENSORS JOURNAL, VOL. 14, NO. 8, AUGUST 2014, Page:2864-2871.
10. E. J. Rouse, L. M. Mooney, and H. M. Herr, "Clutchable series-elastic actuator: implications for prosthetic knee design," International Journal of Robotics Research, vol. 33, no. 13, pp. 1611–1625, 2014.

11. R. Metts, Disability issues, trends and recommendations for the World Bank, Washington, DC (2000).
12. Census of India, Disabled population by type of disability, age, sex and type, Registrar General Office, New Delhi (2001).
13. Francis, P. R., Richman, N. M. & Patterson, P. (1998). Injuries in the sport of racewalking. Journal of Athletic Training, 33(2), 122–129.
14. Chumanov, E. S., Heiderscheit, B. C. & Thelen D. G. (2011). Hamstring musculotendon dynamics during stance and swing phases of high-speed running. Medicine and Science in Sports and Exercise, 43(3), pp.525-532.
15. Todorov E and Jordan MI. Optimal feedback control as a theory of motor coordination. Nat Neurosci 2002; 5: 1226–1235.
16. Berniker M, Jarc A, Bizzi E, et al. Simplified and effective motor control based on muscle synergies to exploit musculoskeletal dynamics. Proc Natl Acad Sci USA 2009.
17. Marchal-Crespo L and Reinkensmeyer DJ. Review of control strategies for robotic movement training after neurologic injury. J Neuroeng Rehabil 2009; 6: 20.
18. Krishnan C, Ranganathan R, Kantak SS, et al. Active robotic training improves locomotor function in a stroke survivor. J Neuroeng Rehabil 2012; 9: 57.
19. Krishnan C, Ranganathan R, Dhaher YY, et al. A pilot study on the feasibility of robot-aided leg motor training to facilitate active participation. PLoS One 2013; 8: e77370.
20. Hussain S, Xie SQ and Liu G. Robot-assisted treadmill training: mechanisms and training strategies. Med Eng Phys 2011; 33: 527–533.
21. Schmidt H, Hesse S, Bernhardt R, et al. HapticWalker – a novel haptic foot device. ACM Trans Appl Percept 2005; 2: 166–180.
22. Schmidt H, Werner C, Bernhardt R, et al. Gait rehabilitation machines based on programmable footplates. J Neuroeng Rehabil 2007; 4: 2.
23. Nielsen JB. How we walk: central control of muscle activity during human walking. Neuroscientist 2003; 9: 195–204.
24. Herr HM, Grabowski AM. Bionic ankle–foot prosthesis normalises walking gait for persons with leg amputation. Proc R Soc B Biol Sci. 2012;279:457–64.
25. Au SK, Herr H, Weber J, Martinez-Villalpando EC. Powered ankle–foot prosthesis for the improvement of amputee ambulation. In: Annual international conference of the IEEE Engineering in

Medicine and Biology — proceedings. New York: Inst. of Elec. And Elec. Eng. Computer Society; 2007. p. 3020–26.
26. Ružicka E, Jankovic JJ. Disorders of gait. In: Jankovic JJ, Tolosa E, editors. Parkinson's disease and movement disorders, 4th ed. Philadelphia: Lippincott, Williams and Wilkins; 2002. pp. 409–29.
27. Juneau, P., Lemaire, E. D., Bavec, A., Burger, H., & Baddour, N. (2022). Automated step detection with 6-minute walk test smartphone sensors signals for fall risk classification in lower limb amputees. PLOS Digital Health, 1(8), e0000088.
28. Griffiths, B., Diment, L., & Granat, M. H. (2021). A machine learning classification model for monitoring the daily physical behaviour of lower-limb amputees. Sensors, 21(22), 7458.
29. Pergolini, A., Livolsi, C., Trigili, E., Chen, B., Giovacchini, F., Forner-Cordero, A., ... & Vitiello, N. (2022). Real-time locomotion recognition algorithm for an active pelvis orthosis to assist lower-limb amputees. IEEE Robotics and Automation Letters, 7(3), 7487-7494.
30. Murray, R., Mendez, J., Gabert, L., Fey, N. P., Liu, H., & Lenzi, T. (2022). Ambulation Mode Classification of Individuals with Transfemoral Amputation through A-Mode Sonomyography and Convolutional Neural Networks. Sensors, 22(23), 9350.
31. Marasco, P. D., Hebert, J. S., Sensinger, J. W., Beckler, D. T., Thumser, Z. C., Shehata, A. W., ... & Wilson, K. R. (2021). Neurorobotic fusion of prosthetic touch, kinesthesia, and movement in bionic upper limbs promotes intrinsic brain behaviours. Science Robotics, 6(58), eabf3368.
32. Kok, M., Hol, J. D., & Schön, T. B. (2017). Using inertial sensors for position and orientation estimation. arXiv preprint arXiv:1704.06053.
33. Agostini, V., Ghislieri, M., Rosati, S., Balestra, G., & Knaflitz, M. (2020). Surface electromyography applied to gait analysis: How to improve its impact in clinics? Frontiers in neurology, 994.
34. Daines, K. J., Baddour, N., Burger, H., Bavec, A., & Lemaire, E. D. (2021). Fall risk classification for people with lower extremity amputations using random forests and smartphone sensor features from a 6-minute walk test. PLoS one, 16(4), e0247574.
35. Khan, A. T., Khajuria, A., Mukherjee, B., & Joshi, D. (2023). A classification framework for investigating neural correlates of the limit of stability during weight-shifting in lower limb amputees. Neurocomputing, 524, 84-94.

36. Liang, F. Y., Gao, F., Cao, J., Law, S. W., & Liao, W. H. (2022). Gait synergy analysis and modelling on amputees and stroke patients for lower limb assistive devices. Sensors, 22(13), 4814.
37. Stolyarov, R., Carney, M., & Herr, H. (2020). Accurate heuristic terrain prediction in powered lower-limb prostheses using onboard sensors. IEEE Transactions on Biomedical Engineering, 68(2), 384–392.
38. Su, B. Y., Wang, J., Liu, S. Q., Sheng, M., Jiang, J., & Xiang, K. (2019). A CNN-based method for intent recognition using inertial measurement units and intelligent lower limb prosthesis. IEEE Transactions on Neural Systems and Rehabilitation Engineering, 27(5), 1032-1042.
39. Marcos Mazon, D., Groefsema, M., Schomaker, L. R., & Carloni, R. (2022). IMU-Based Classification of Locomotion Modes, Transitions, and Gait Phases with Convolutional Recurrent Neural Networks. Sensors, 22(22), 8871.
40. Karakish, M., Fouz, M. A., & ELsawaf, A. (2022). Gait Trajectory Prediction on an Embedded Microcontroller Using Deep Learning. Sensors, 22(21), 8441.
41. de Mendonça Mesquita, E., Rodrigues, A. P., de Oliveira Andrade, A., & Vieira, M. F. (2020). Classification of Lower Limb Amputees Gait Using Machine Learning Algorithms. In VIII Latin American Conference on Biomedical Engineering and XLII National Conference on Biomedical Engineering: Proceedings of CLAIB-CNIB 2019, October 2-5, 2019, Cancún, México (pp. 950-954). Springer International Publishing.

CHAPTER 10

WIRELESS SHAPE MEMORY NITINOL STENT

NUSRAT HASSAN KHAN[1], ANG YONG XIAN,[1] MARIATUL RAWDHAH AHMAD FUAAD,[1] MOHAMED SULTAN MOHAMED ALI[1,2]

[1]Faculty of Electrical Engineering, Universiti Teknologi Malaysia, 81310 UTM Johor Bahru, Johor, Malaysia
[2]Department of Electrical Engineering, College of Engineering, Qatar University, Doha, Qatar

Abstract: This chapter discusses the development of an intelligent stent for atherosclerosis treatment, which includes a wireless monitoring mechanism and expansion feature after deployment. The problem of blood vessels re-narrowing following percutaneous transluminal angioplasty and various stents designed to address this issue is also discussed in detail. This chapter focuses on developing a nitinol stent with wireless capabilities for re-expansion and pressure sensing. The fabrication process and ex-vivo testing are described, and the stent was successfully expanded wirelessly using radio frequency signals, resulting in a 17% increase in diameter. Overall, the results of this study are promising for the proposed design and application of stents in managing atherosclerosis.

Keywords: *Atherosclerosis, Stents, Wireless, Actuator, Shape Memory Alloy, Nitinol.*

1. INTRODUCTION

The COVID-19 outbreak has spotlighted the need for remote medical monitoring systems. With the increased risk of contagion and the need for reduced in-person appointments, wireless monitoring systems have become vital in treating long-term health issues. An area where wireless monitoring can have a substantial impact is in using shape memory active nitinol stents for blood vessel revitalisation. Atherosclerosis is when the blood vessels become narrowed due to plaque build-up on their walls. This might result in restricted circulation to specific areas of the anatomy, leading to cardiac conditions such as chest pain or myocardial infarction. One treatment option is percutaneous transluminal angioplasty (PTA), which involves using a balloon-tipped catheter to widen the narrowed blood vessels and restore blood flow. However, this procedure may also result in a complication referred to as restenosis, blood vessel re-narrowing that occurs in the aftermath of PTA [1]. Therefore, a tube with a net-like structure compatible with a living body familiarised as a stent is frequently inserted with balloon dilation to substantially broaden and stabilise the blood venules to thwart this complication.

There have been multiple advancements in stenting techniques following the advent of bare-metal stents (BMSs), including self-expanding stents (SESs), drug-eluting stents (DESs), and bioresorbable stents (BRSs). A stent must exert adequate radial force to act as a scaffold and keep the vessel open. BMSs, typically made of stainless steel, are inserted using catheters with expandable balloons, also called balloon-extending stents (BESs). However, even though BMSs have successfully improved the existing technology, vessel narrowing is still on an upward trend due to gradual tissue growth within the stent. This is known as re-narrowing of the stent and is observed in 30% of cases within six months. [2]. Sometimes the term "in-stent restenosis" (ISR) refers to the same condition. [3]. Stents were created with a coating containing cell growth inhibitors that are liberated to impede or decrease the tissue formation within the stent, thereby averting re-narrowing to address the high stent re-narrowing rate attributed to BMSs.

The initial making of stents coated with cell growth inhibitors utilised sirolimus as the inhibiting agent. This reduced the stent re-narrowing to 6% but caused an uptick in blood clot formation, known as stent thrombosis (ST). Alarmingly, this higher ST incidence is dangerous and may cause fatal complications associated with heart attack and death [4 - 6]. Consequently, to address this issue, later versions of stents coated with cell growth inhibitors were created to abate delayed clotting within the stent and impede the growth of the inner lining tissue simultaneously [7]. This was accomplished by substituting the traditional stainless-steel material employed in the stents' initial iteration coated with cell growth inhibitors for cobalt-chromium or platinum chromium, resulting in stents of less thickness. Besides, everolimus or zotarolimus was used as a new drug replacing sirolimus. Despite that, using permanent polymers for drug elution is still associated with stent thrombogenicity [8].

Another iteration has been created utilising materials that disintegrate or dissolve over time to address the thrombogenicity problem with stents coated with permanent polymers. The dissolvable or bioresorbable stents (BRSs) are divided into two categories based on what they are made of – dissolvable polymers and bioresorbable metals. Stents constructed using dissolvable polymers such as poly-lactide can degrade over time due to hydrolysis. However, they are not as sturdy as metal stents and can generate a reaction in the venule's inner lining. To circumvent these limitations, stents made from bioresorbable metals such as magnesium and zinc, commonly found in the human body, have been developed. These stents provide similar rigidity and firmness to stainless steel stents, but the dissolution process is completed within 6 to 24 months. Yet, there are still issues to address with these stents, such as compatibility and resistance to magnesium stents corrosion and the rapid rate of zinc stents dissolution, which may affect the scaffold function during vessel healing [9, 10].

Like BES, SES also operates on a self-expanding mechanism where Shape Memory Effect (SME) plays a crucial role. SME has been demonstrated in several biomedical applications [11, 12]. In contrast to stents that provide outward force through malleable change during positioning and expansion of narrowed lesions, Self-Expanding Stents utilise the extraordinary springiness of Shape Memory Alloys to exert outward force. **Figure 1** compares the operating principle of BES and SES. **Figure 1a** shows a pre-crimped BES that is then inflated with a balloon, causing it to reach its intended size. As the balloon inflates, it causes the BES to undergo plastic deformation. On the other hand, **Figure 1b** shows a Nitinol stent that, due to its high radial force, is compressed and held within a retractable delivery sheath before being placed in the body, which allows it to withstand being squeezed by the artery constriction after it has been deployed. The SES exerts a constant low force to expand and open a blockage until it reaches its maximum size. Nitinol is biocompatible and one of medical implants' most used shape memory alloys. The benefits of super-elastic hysteresis allow Nitinol stents to have a powerful radial resistance and low long-term outward force. These stents can be compressed and held within a sheath with retractable delivery before implementation and withstand compression from narrowed blood vessels after disposition. The stent keeps applying a low, ongoing, outward force, widening the specific venule until it reaches its largest size. This enables the stent to reach its pre-determined shape without significant contraction as time passes. [13].

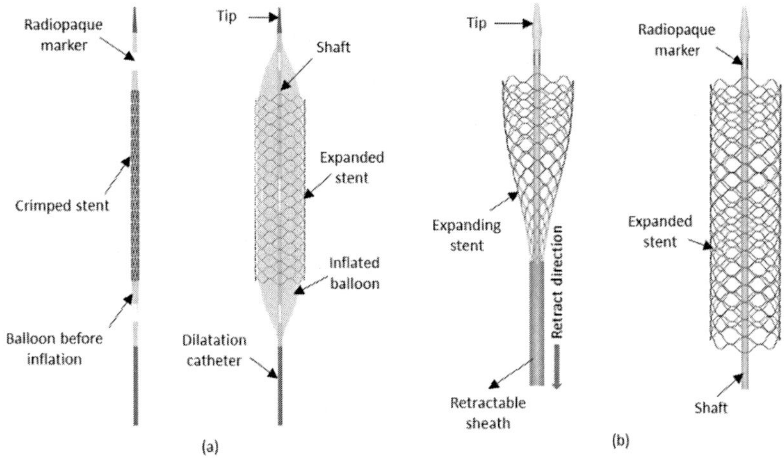

Figure 1 Operating principle of a) BES and b) SES.

Stents have limitations, such as ISR occurrence and the inability to detect stenosis recurrence without additional procedures such as angiography or ultrasound [14]. Smart devices using the MEMS approach have been developed to wirelessly monitor restenosis. An advanced device utilising a resonant circuit with an LC configuration in a closed-loop layout has been created with various transducer capabilities, including wireless blood pressure measurement and remote transmission capabilities. [15, 16]. Supplementary studies have created a helical stent of stainless steel with a micro-pressure sensor and wireless communication capabilities to detect restenosis. The stent also has a wireless heating feature for hyperthermia treatment [17, 18]. Regardless, this type of stent is not fully effective in protecting against in-stent restenosis.

This chapter introduces a new helical stent that incorporates a Nitinol alloy with thermo-responsive properties and a sensor for measuring pressure to address the issue of restenosis, as depicted in **Figure 2**. **Figure 2a** details the stent's installation principle. The device includes an LC circuit as part of its architecture, which can monitor changes in artery pressure via continuous remote monitoring. The helical stent made of Nitinol alloy is intended as a thermally responsive actuator and allows repeated wireless stent revascularisation to re-establish circulation in instances of ISR.

Figure 2b illustrates the flow of the concept for wireless monitoring and ISR treatment. The design and properties of the stent were studied using finite element analysis, steps to fabricate the device and thermal characteristics. Afterwards, ex-vivo testing was implemented.

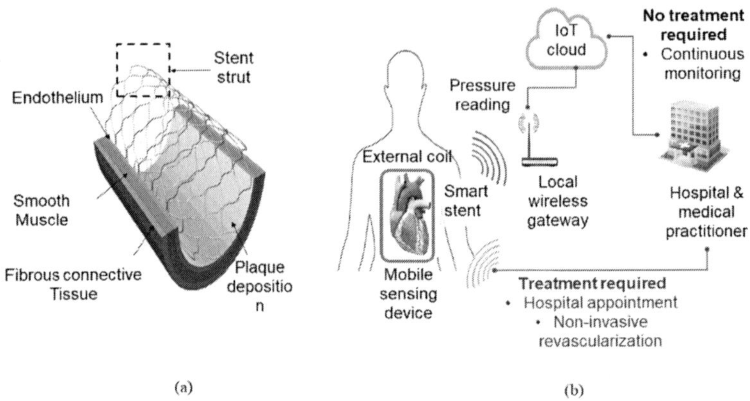

Figure 2 Biomedical a) stent deployment in the lesioned artery and b) potential advancements in remote monitoring.

2. WORKING PRINCIPLE

Nitinol is a special alloy with exceptional resilience and the ability to return to its original shape. It exists in two solid phases: austenitic and martensitic, characterised by the transformation between the two phases. Super-elasticity (SE) refers to Nitinol's ability to return to its original shape without permanent deformation triggered by stress-induced mechanisms. Shape memory effect (SME) refers to Nitinol's ability to remember a pre-determined shape, triggered by temperature-induced mechanisms and achieved through thermal-annealing and cooling processes. Nitinol is commonly used in stents, as depicted in **Figure 3**, which are medical devices that widen narrowed or obstructed blood vessels.

Figure 3 demonstrates the intended device's performance mechanism, which can treat ISR by inflating remotely in several junctures. **Figure 3a** pictures vessel compression due to the accumulation of unwanted clots hindering the body's regular circulation. When conducting percutaneous transluminal angioplasty, the stent is placed at the lesion with the aid of a catheter [13,14]. Then as per the stent's physical feature, whether the balloon blows up or self-expands, it prepares to remove the undesired constriction (**Figure 3b**). **Figure 3c** shows the installed stent made of Nitinol, a shape memory alloy after enlargement.

The proposed stent works based on a microelectromechanical system that can read the pressure change in the venule. Calculating the pressure analyses the ISR's condition (**Figure 3d).** When the vessel compression is detected again within the stent, and the situation needs to be taken care of, a radio frequency (RF) signal is introduced that adjusts itself to the resonance frequency of the nitinol structure, and this re-expands the system generating heat [19]. Blood flow is restored as the vessel is opened by the implanted stent without requiring a second surgery, as pointed out in **Figure 3e.** The relationship between the resonant frequency f_R, Capacitance, C and Inductance, L is given by;

$$f_R = 1/\left(2\pi\sqrt{LC}\right) \qquad (1)$$

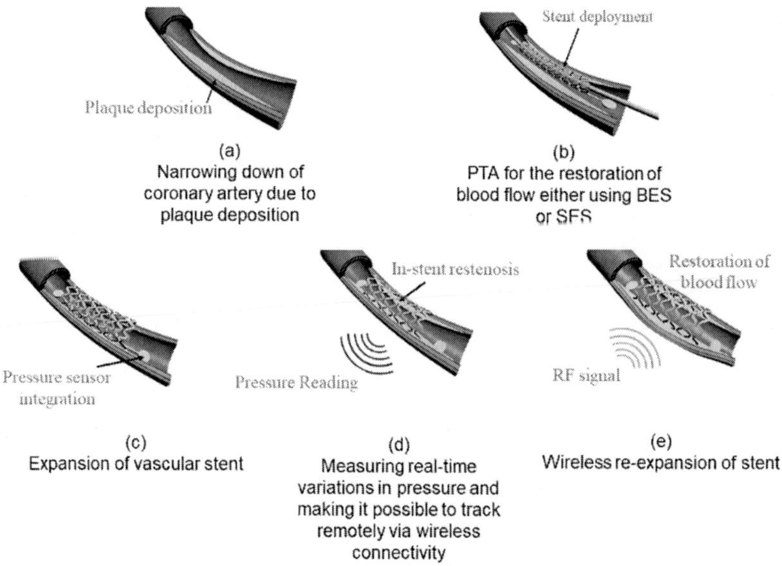

Figure 3 The fundamental concept of Nitinol stent's mechanism.

3. DESIGN AND SIMULATION

The innovative stent configuration shown in **Figure 4** consists of a nitinol stent with induction properties and a sensor that measures pressure through capacitance, resulting in a resonant circuit. The stent's size and environment determine its inductive properties. This allows for real-time monitoring of the stent's diameter and the pressure within the blood vessel. The pressure sensor, integrated into the stent, measures the pressure changes and sends the data wirelessly to a remote monitoring device. This active design allows for early restenosis detection, which is the blood vessel re-narrowing after stent implantation and permits subsequent wireless stent recanalisation to improve blood circulation. In addition, the active stent design provides a more reliable and efficient method for monitoring stent performance and preventing restenosis than traditional passive stents.

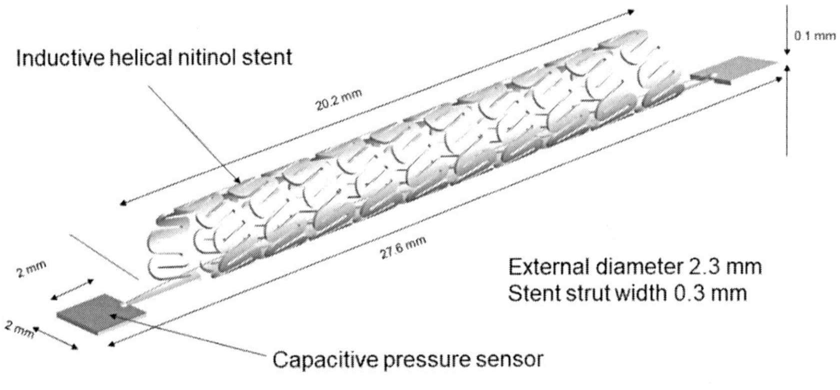

Figure 4 Designed nitinol stent.

The equation gives the formula to determine the capacitance of a parallel-plate capacitor:

$$C = \varepsilon_0 \varepsilon_r(T) \frac{A}{d} \quad (2)$$

The permittivity of free space ε_0 and the relative permittivity of the dielectric material $\varepsilon_r(T)$ changes with temperature. The area, A, and the thickness, d, of the dielectric layer are all factors used in the capacitance calculation. The relative magnetic permeability of the medium μ

represents the magnetic permeability measurement of the environment surrounding the object,

$$\mu_r = 1 + X_m \quad (3)$$

The change in magnetic susceptibility, X_m, is a function of the temperature and depends on the material's properties. Tissue and liquids like saline and oxygenated blood are considered diamagnetic, meaning their effect on the resonant frequency is minimal, similar to a vacuum. Nevertheless, the resonant frequency can be impacted by the material's temperature-dependent electrical permittivity [20, 21]. To achieve better resonant frequency accuracy, measuring it experimentally at a relevant temperature is recommended. This eventually allows the change in resonant frequency with different stent diameters to be observed. **Figure 5a** displays the software replication results of the inductance measurements on the stent's various forms. Observe that the stent's expansion is directly proportional to inductance. The active stent's thermomechanical actuation is connected to the hysteresis feature of Nitinol's one-way SME. Figure 5b illustrates the thermomechanical behaviour of a Nitinol sample. A notable loop in the graph indicates a full-phase transformation between the martensitic and austenitic phases. The smaller loop in the graph represents the hysteretic behaviour of Nitinol during repeated thermal loading. The numbering in the figure illustrates the transformation order during cooling and heating, and this type of loading path is used for the Nitinol active stent.

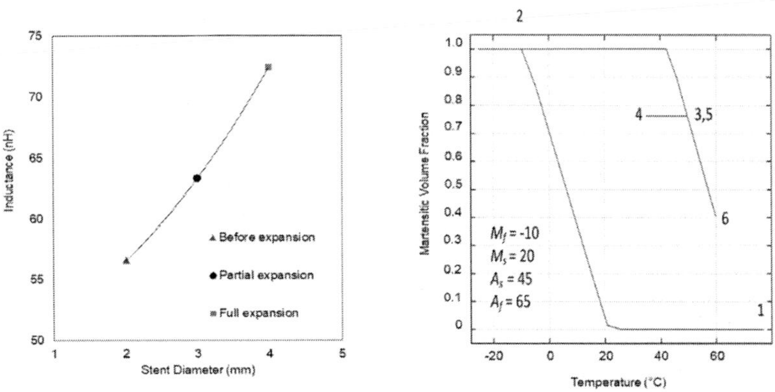

(a) (b)

Figure 5 a) The simulation graph of stent diameter vs Inductance b) Temperature vs Martensitic Volume Fraction.

4. FABRICATION

Figure 6 illustrates the fabrication process of a nitinol active stent. The first step involves using a wire-electro-discharge-machining technique to cut a sheet of Nitinol with an approximate width of 100 μm into a serpentine shape with a built-in cavity for a capacitive pressure sensor (**Figure 6a**). This engineered structure is then wrapped around and fixed to a steel rod attachment with an approximate diameter of 5 mm to achieve a broader diameter range. Then, it is heated at 45°C in a furnace for 45 minutes to set its shape (**Figure 6b**). After heating, the stent's surface removes the blue oxide layer by etching to smoothen the surface (**Figure 6c**).

Figure 6d shows the stent's size in its initial state and after being compressed onto an implement with a size of 2 mm. The device is then crammed into a miniature structure with residual tension for re-expansion when excited. When the coil was compressed, the number of turns nearly doubled. A capacitive pressure sensor is then created by covering the cavity area with a dielectric layer made of polydimethylsiloxane (PDMS) and a fine imparting stainless-steel layer, as shown in **Figure 6e**. Finally, an LC resonant circuit was created by utilising a conductive silver epoxy and a silver wire made of silver to connect the device and the sensor to measure capacitance. This circuit was then allowed to cure for 24 hours at ambient temperature. The device is then coated with an electrical insulation layer of around three μm extent for protection, and the final product is shown in **Figure 6f**. Finally, **Figure 7a** presents a picture of the produced active nitinol stent.

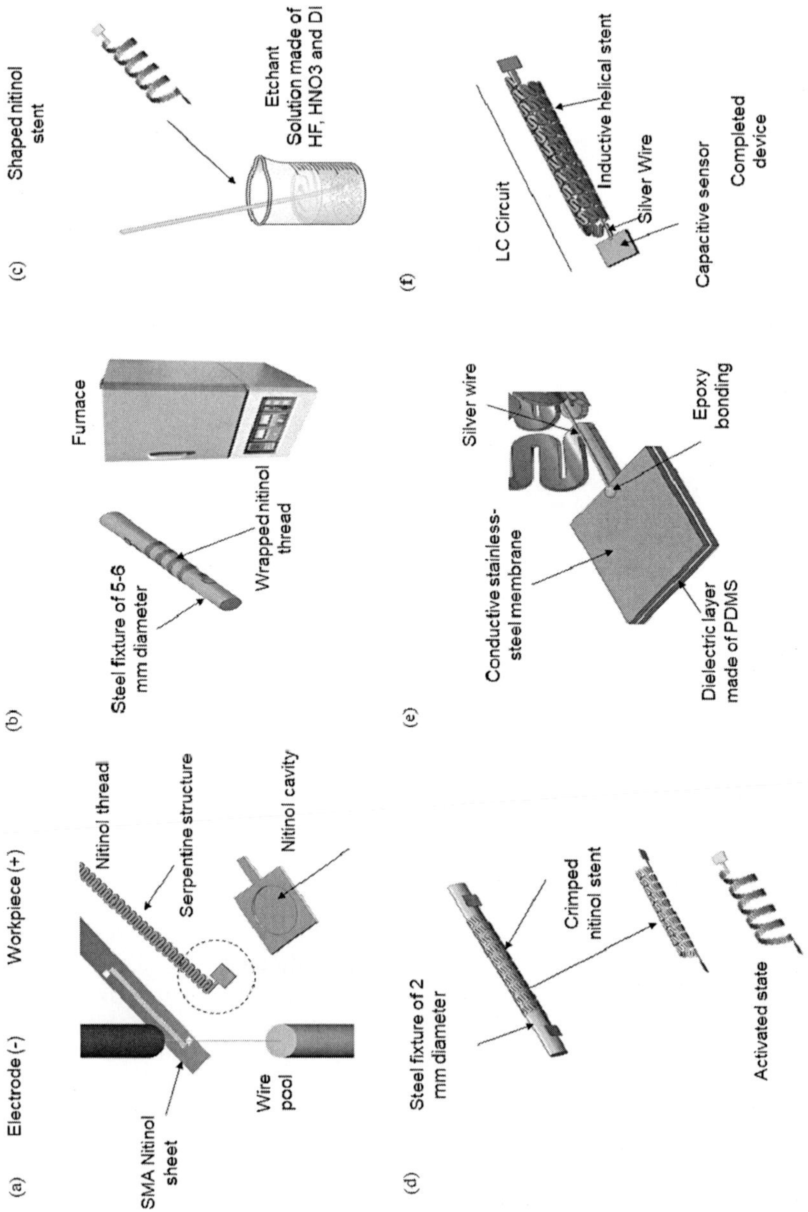

Figure 6 Fabrication steps of Nitinol active state

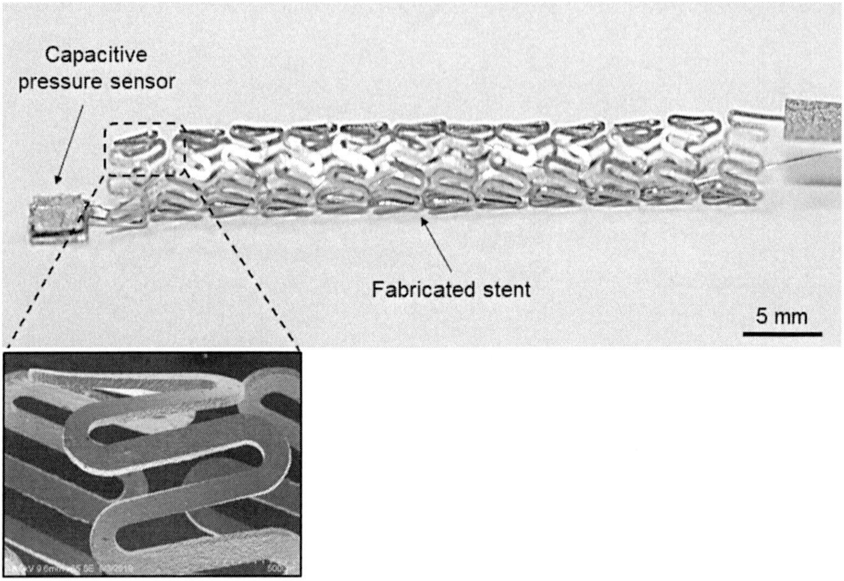

Figure 7 a) Fabrication of shape memory active nitinol stent.

5. RESULTS AND DISCUSSION

This section presents and examines the experiment outcomes, emphasising the heat and time reactions of the nitinol active stent when activated wirelessly. Also assessed is the stent's outside-the-body effectiveness using a living organism's blood vessel model.

5.1 Thermal and Temporal Characterisation

The device was inserted into synthetic rubber tubing and activated using radio waves. It was initially activated at a frequency of 315 MHz and power of 11.7 Watts until it reached full activation at 230 MHz and 29.5 Watts. **Figure 8** shows the thermal images of the stent during this process. There were issues with thermographic emissivity due to the reflective properties of the synthetic rubber tubing and the stent. These were addressed by removing a portion of the synthetic rubber tubing to eliminate its infrared radiation shielding effect and by covering the nitinol device with a material that eliminated the emissivity problem and protected it against the unwanted electric shock. Camera images also show the device's progressive expansion inside a transparent silicon tube with a diameter of 3.5 mm.

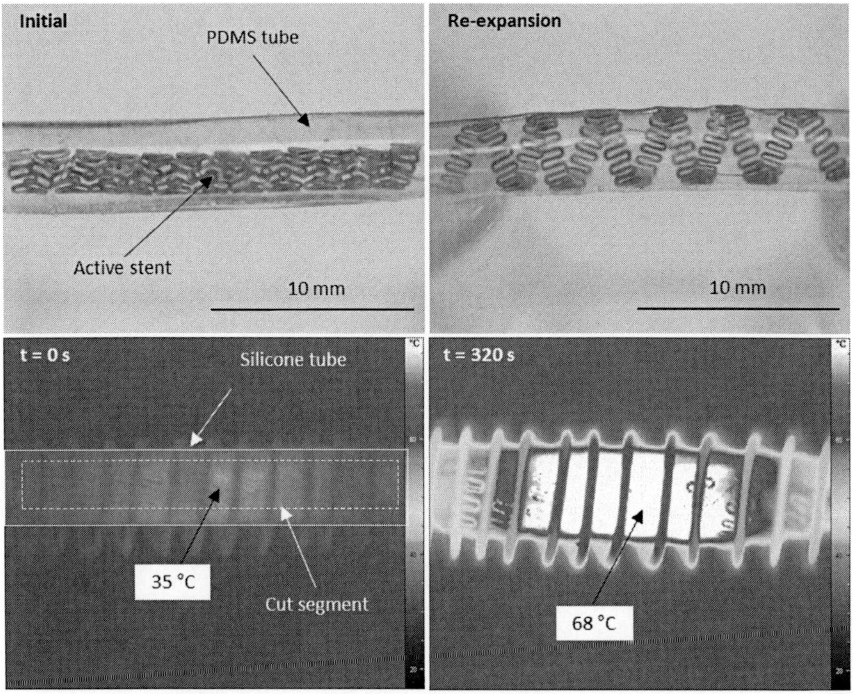

Figure 8 Stent images procured from digital and thermal cameras, respectively.

In the initial state, the size of the stent (**Figure 8**) was expanded to 3.2 mm by utilising a powerful radio frequency signal of 315 MHz with an output of 11.7 W for 220 seconds. The frequency was altered to 270 MHz to align with the frequency of the partly inflated stent by increasing the radio frequency output to continue expanding the stent. At the 320-second mark, the stent was extended to a mean diameter of 4.2 mm. The typical thermal distribution was stimulated during the initial expansion at 315 MHz (**Figure 9a**). The central portion of the stent registers a higher temperature, suggesting that the wireless resonant heating begins in the middle and subsequently spreads to both the proximal and distal regions.

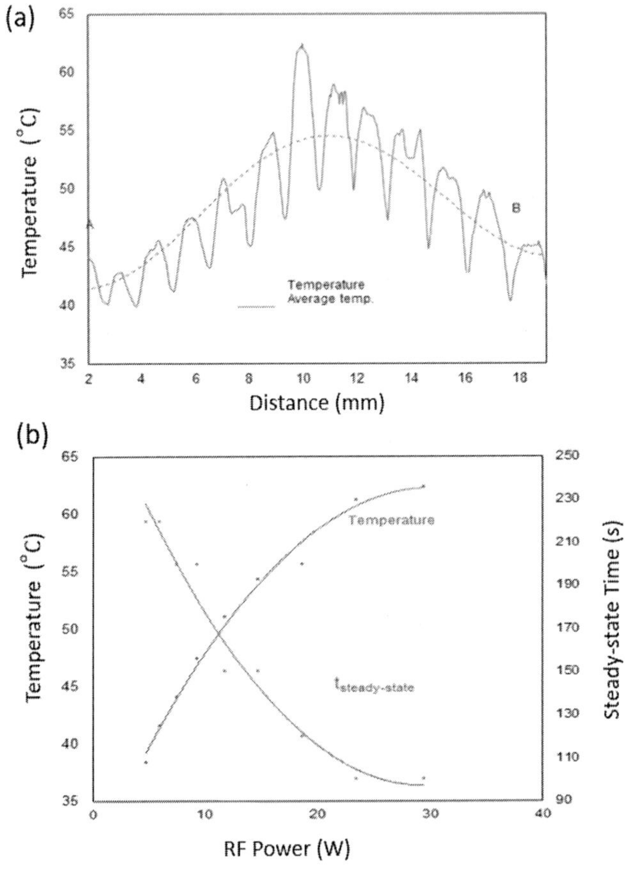

Figure 9 a) Thermal energy distribution during actuation. (b) The relationship between stent temperature and steady state time.

Furthermore, **Figure 9b** illustrates a temperature increase while the stent is enlarged, demonstrating uniform heat transfer throughout the device. Subsequently, the frequency was altered to 230 MHz. Utilising a higher radio frequency leads to a shorter duration for the stent's temperature to become stable. This implies that the radio frequency power, external field frequency, and activation duration must be refined to impede a temperature rise during stent enlargement.

5.2 Ex-vivo study

A study was conducted using an active stent implanted in a heart obtained from a deer. The stent was inserted through the aorta and guided to the left circumflex artery using a guidewire using an endoscope. The left circumflex artery segment, with a standard internal measurement of 2.9 mm, positioned 25 mm from the left primary coronary opening, was used as a stenotic lesion. The active stent was then advanced along the guidewire path to reach the lesion. **Figure 10** shows the detailed ex-vivo characterisation step by step.

The dynamic implant was inserted into the deer's heart. The catheter was extracted after the deer's vessel was embedded with a dynamic implant. The stented area within the cervine heart was examined using an X-ray fluoroscopy system, as shown in **Figure 10a**. Initially, an external coil with a tuned external field frequency that matches the resonant frequency was used to expand the implanted active stent through resonant inductive coupling. The external coil was positioned for wireless electro-thermomechanical expansion at the LCX lesion site on the cervine heart. In the beginning, the active stent's average diameter was 2.4 mm. The dimension of the dynamic implant increased by 17% from its starting point when activated by a radio frequency power of 18.6 W, resulting in a measurement of 2.8 mm, which was close to the standard internal measurement of the coronary artery's secondary branch. **Figure 10b** shows the radiographic images of the dynamic implant in its inactive state and after expansion. The strut went from crimped to an enlarged profile when the active stent was wirelessly triggered.

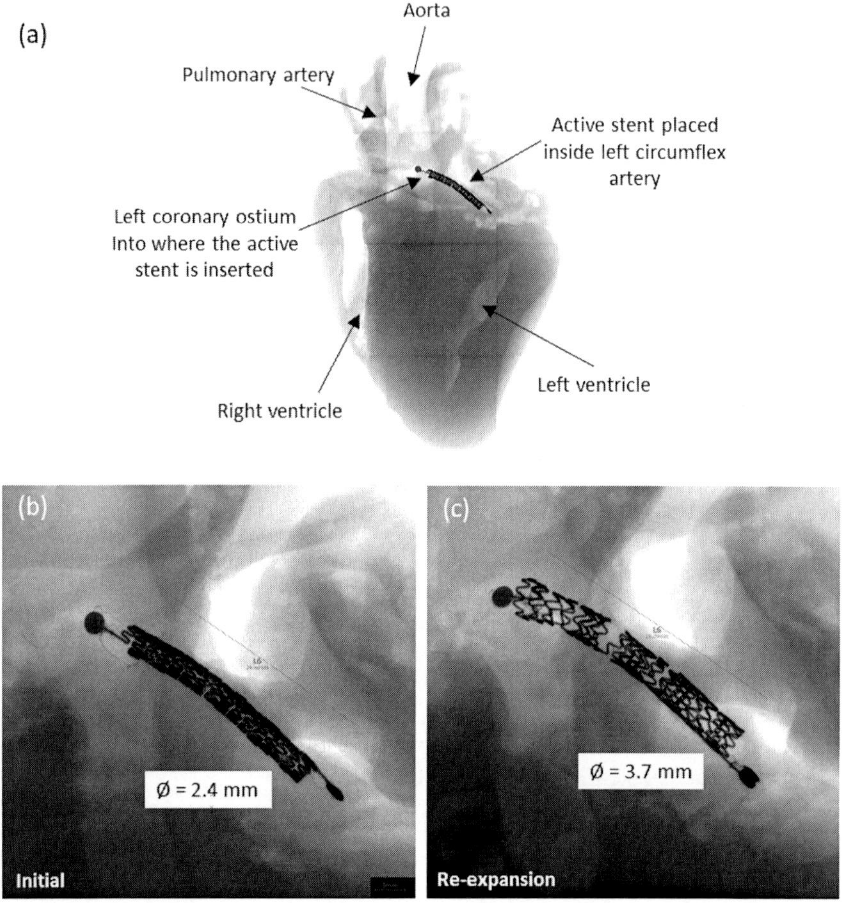

Figure 10 a) Camera image of stent insertion. (b) X-Ray image of the compressed stent. (c) X-ray image of the activated or expanded stent

CONCLUSION

A brand-new SMA Nitinol type active stent was demonstrated using wireless monitoring and revascularisation characteristics. Wireless re-vascularised was made possible by utilising Nitinol's shape recovery feature and the spiral design for wireless activation. Remote monitoring was made possible by measuring the variation in resonant frequency shift. The COVID and post-COVID eras would do well to consider this wireless capability. The nitinol active stent's wireless testing's thermal and temporal responses were characterised. The dynamic stent with a measurement of 2 mm was stretched to 3.2 mm and then to 4.2 mm by increasing the radio frequency power to 29.5 W for 100 s by utilising a radio frequency power of 11.7 W at 315 MHz for a duration of 220 s.

Following the first enhancement, the stent's dimension increased by 60% from its contracted state, and after the second enhancement, it increased by 31.25% from its partially enhanced state. During the laboratory trial using a removed organ, the implant expanded by 17% from its initial size when activated with a radio frequency energy of 18.6 W. To further expand the implant by 32% from its partially expanded state, the amount of radio frequency energy required was increased to 46.7 W. The increase was attributed to the thicker tissue layer and the decreased electromagnetic field when a gap existed between the external coil and the implant.

The monolithic active stent design will be improved in the next study. A live animal test is necessary to evaluate the stent's practicality and effectiveness in real-world conditions. The procedure's suitability for treating blood vessels re-narrowing without invasive surgery depends on the Nitinol alloy selection that is responsive to the appropriate temperature range similar to a human body.

REFERENCES

[1] F. Alfonso and J. Cuesta, "The therapeutic dilemma of recurrent in-stent restenosis," *Circ Cardiovasc Interv*, vol. 11, no. 8, p. 7109, 2018, DoI: 10.1161/CIRCINTERVENTIONS.118.007109.

[2] A. Gaspardone and F. Versaci, "Coronary stenting and inflammation.," *Am J Cardiol*, vol. 96, no. 12 A, pp. 65–70, 2005, DoI: 10.1016/J.AMJCARD.2005.09.064.

[3] Y. X. Ang, M. Sultan, and M. Ali, "Inductive Helical Stent for Wireless Revascularization: Finite Element Analysis," *ELEKTRIKA- Journal of Electrical Engineering*, vol. 20, no. 2–2, pp. 20–24, Sep. 2021, Accessed: Jan. 17, 2023. [Online]. Available: https://elektrika.utm.my/index.php/ELEKTRIKA_Journal/article/view/302

[4] I. Akin *et al.*, "Second- and third-generation drug-eluting coronary stents: progress and safety," *Herz*, vol. 36, no. 3, pp. 190–197, 2011, DoI: 10.1007/S00059-011-3458-Z.

[5] C. Stettler *et al.*, "Outcomes associated with drug-eluting and bare-metal stents: a collaborative network meta-analysis," *Lancet*, vol.

370, no. 9591, pp. 937–948, Sep 2007, DoI: 10.1016/S0140-6736(07)61444-5.
[6] A. Schömig *et al.*, “A meta-analysis of 16 randomised trials of sirolimus-eluting stents versus paclitaxel-eluting stents in patients with coronary artery disease,” *J Am Coll Cardiol*, vol. 50, no. 14, pp. 1373–1380, Oct 2007, DoI: 10.1016/J.JACC.2007.06.047.
[7] M. Joner *et al.*, “Endothelial Cell Recovery Between Comparator Polymer-Based Drug-Eluting Stents,” *J Am Coll Cardiol*, vol. 52, no. 5, pp. 333–342, Jul. 2008, DoI: 10.1016/J.JACC.2008.04.030.
[8] K. D. Rizas and J. Mehilli, “Stent Polymers: Do They Make a Difference?,” *Circ Cardiovasc Interv*, vol. 9, no. 6, Jun 2016, DoI: 10.1161/CIRCINTERVENTIONS.115.002943.
[9] J. S. Bergström and D. Hayman, “An Overview of Mechanical Properties and Material Modeling of Polylactide (PLA) for Medical Applications,” *Ann Biomed Eng*, vol. 44, no. 2, pp. 330–340, Feb 2016, DoI: 10.1007/S10439-015-1455-8/TABLES/2.
[10] H. Jinnouchi, S. Torii, A. Sakamoto, F. D. Kolodgie, R. Virmani, and A. v. Finn, “Fully bioresorbable vascular scaffolds: lessons learned and future directions,” *Nat Rev Cardiol*, vol. 16, no. 5, pp. 286–304, May 2019, DoI: 10.1038/S41569-018-0124-7.
[11] M. R. A. Kadir, D. E. O. Dewi, M. N. Jamaludin, M. Nafea, and M. S. M. Ali, “A multi-segmented shape memory alloy-based actuator system for endoscopic applications,” *Sensors and Actuators A: Physical,* vol. 296, pp. 92-100, 2019.
[12] A. AbuZaiter, M. Nafea, A. A. M. Faudzi, S. Kazi, and M. S. M. Ali, “Thermomechanical behaviour of bulk NiTi shape-memory-alloy microactuators based on bimorph actuation,” *Microsystem Technologies,* vol. 22, no. 8, pp. 2125-2131, 2016.
[13] Y. X. Ang, A. Z. M. Khudzari, and M. S. M. Ali, “Non-Invasive Treatment for Coronary In-Stent Restenosis via Wireless Revascularization With Nitinol Active Stent,” *IEEE Trans Biomed Eng*, vol. 68, no. 12, pp. 3681–3689, Dec 2021, DoI: 10.1109/TBME.2021.3082172.
[14] Y. X. Ang, F. A. M. Ghazali, and M. S. M. Ali, “Micromachined Shape Memory Alloy Active Stent with Wireless Monitoring and Re-Expansion Features,” *Proceedings of the IEEE International Conference on Micro Electro Mechanical Systems (MEMS)*, vol. 2020-January, pp. 396–399, Jan 2020, DoI: 10.1109/MEMS46641.2020.9056379.
[15] K. Takahata, Y. B. Gianchandani, and K. D. Wise, “Micromachined antenna stents and cuffs for monitoring intraluminal pressure and

flow," *Journal of Microelectromechanical Systems*, vol. 15, no. 5, pp. 1289–1298, Oct 2006, DoI: 10.1109/JMEMS.2006.880229.
[16] A. R. Mohammadi, M. S. Mohamed Ali, D. Lappin, C. Schlosser, and K. Takahata, "Inductive antenna stent: design, fabrication and characterisation," *Journal of Micromechanics and Microengineering*, vol. 23, no. 2, p. 025015, Jan 2013, DoI: 10.1088/0960-1317/23/2/025015.
[17] Y. Yi, J. Chen, M. Selvaraj, Y. Hsiang, and K. Takahata, "Wireless Hyperthermia Stent System for Restenosis Treatment and Testing With Swine Model," *IEEE Trans Biomed Eng*, vol. 67, no. 4, pp. 1097–1104, Apr 2020, DoI: 10.1109/TBME.2019.2929265.
[18] X. Ji, J. Zheng, R. Yang, W. Kainz, and J. Chen, "Evaluations of the MRI RF-Induced Heating for Helical Stents under a 1.5T MRI System," *IEEE Trans Electromagn Compat*, vol. 61, no. 1, pp. 57–64, Feb 2019, DoI: 10.1109/TEMC.2017.2785180.
[19] P. S. Chee, M. Nafea, P. L. Leow, and M. S. M. Ali, "Thermal analysis of wirelessly powered thermo-pneumatic micropump based on planar LC circuit," Journal of Mechanical Science and Technology, vol. 30, no. 6, pp. 2659-2665, 2016.
[20] P. V. Prasad, R. R. Edelman, and F. H. Epstein, "Non-invasive evaluation of intrarenal oxygenation with BOLD MRI," *circulation*, vol. 94, no. 12, pp. 3271–3275, 1996, DoI: 10.1161/01.CIR.94.12.3271.
[21] J. F. Schenck, "The role of magnetic susceptibility in magnetic resonance imaging: MRI magnetic compatibility of the first and second kinds," *Med Phys*, vol. 23, no. 6, pp. 815–850, 1996, DoI: 10.1118/1.597854.

CHAPTER 11

TISSUE ENGINEERING AND REGENERATIVE MEDICINE-BASED STRATEGIES FOR COVID-19 TREATMENT

RUCHI MISHRA TIWARI[1*], ASHWINI KUMAR[2]

[1]Symbiosis Centre for Stem Cell Research, Symbiosis International University, Lavale, Maharashtra-412115, India
[2]Biotechnology & Bioinformatics Area, NIIT University, Neemrana, Rajasthan

ABSTRACT

The COVID-19 pandemic has had a distressing impact on the worldwide population, mainly in terms of a substantial number of deaths and deterioration of social and economic conditions. It also led to a significant shift in research focus towards the generation of treatment strategies for COVID-19 disease, which further affected the research and development activities in other areas such as Tissue Engineering and Regenerative Medicine (TERM). On the other hand, TERM-based treatment strategies for COVID-19 formed a promising aspect to looking for a cure rather than managing the infection. Therefore, in this chapter, we discuss the role of TERM-based strategies in developing treatment options for COVID-19 infections through cell-based therapy, mesenchymal stem cell (MSC) exosome-based therapy, *in vitro* models/organoid systems, vaccine technology and small-molecule based therapy. The chapter also discusses the short and long-term ill effects of COVID-19 on the lungs and other organs such as the heart, liver, kidney, etc.

Keywords: *COVID-19, Exosomes, Lungs, Mesenchymal stem cell (MSC), Tissue Engineering and Regenerative Medicine (TERM)*

1. INTRODUCTION

COVID-19 is considered one of the worst pandemics of the past century, with a global death toll reported in the millions. The death toll is further expected to be much more than the reported cases, with 13.2 million and 16.6 million higher numbers estimated for 2020 and 2021, respectively.[1] The pandemic has hit us hard with not only the number of deaths but also the amount of damage it has caused society in the form of economic and social impact. Amongst others, COVID-19 has impacted tissue engineering and regenerative medicine (TERM) by hampering the proper running of research facilities due to various issues such as transportation difficulties, the possibility of COVID-19 infections, lack of supplies, etc. One of the examples is its impact on the field of musculoskeletal tissue engineering, wherein treatment delay for osteoarthritic lesions might lead to an increase in patient number requiring joint replacement in the long run.[2] Other effects can be direct effects such as virus reaching and infecting musculoskeletal tissues, and indirect effects may be due to the ill effects on musculoskeletal tissues due to long periods of being immobile during ICU stays or restricted mobility due to home isolation/lockdown as well as work-from-home or remote working activities.[3] Another major example of the impact of COVID-19 is on cell transplantation therapy, particularly about hematopoietic stem cells. The associated effect mainly includes a lack of donors (especially the uninfected donors), problems related to safe transportation at the donation site, including the need for special permission, and issues with collection, storage (cryopreservation), *in vitro* modification, and *ex vivo* expansion.[4,5] Other than these examples, there have been direct implications in funds drain towards research on COVID-19. Therefore, much of the funding for other research activities, including TERM research, was cut off or redirected towards the research on the COVID-19 pandemic.[3,4] Contrary to the ill effects of COVID-19 on TERM research, this research field has, in return, positively contributed significantly in the form of novel strategies for the management and treatment of the disease. TERM research has not only helped in developing novel treatments for COVID-19 disease but also addresses the long-term ill-effects of this disease (long-COVID) on various organs by coming up with possible solutions. Therefore, this chapter discusses the strategies based on TERM research that have been developed so far.

2. ROLE OF TERM RESEARCH IN GENERATING TREATMENTS FOR THE COVID-19 PANDEMIC

Since the inception of the 21st century, there have been multiple viral outbreaks, such as, in 2003 outbreak of Severe Acute Respiratory Syndrome Coronavirus occurred, followed by the Ebola virus in 2014, Middle Eastern Respiratory Syndrome Coronavirus as well as Zika Virus in 2015, and, the outbreak of Severe Acute Respiratory Syndrome Coronavirus 2 (SARS-CoV-2) virus most recently, i.e., 2019.[6] Therefore, there is a dire need of novel mechanisms at a high priority to handle these outbreaks in the form of robust and reliant treatment strategies.

As a part of TERM approaches, tissue engineering is an exciting option as an interdisciplinary field that relies on the crosstalk between experts in different disciplines, such as chemistry, physics, biology, engineering, medicine, etc., to develop strategies that could reach from the level of laboratory-based research to actual application in clinics in the form of TERM-based products. COVID-19 treatment strategies also require crosstalk between virologists, clinicians, genetic engineers, cell biologists, and many more experts from various disciplines. Therefore, TERM has the potential to come up with strategies that could help in the cure of COVID-19 rather than just managing the infection like in the case of most of the other methods used for COVID-19 treatment.[6,7]

Another application of tissue engineering for COVID-19 treatment could be for the treatment of the organs that get directly and indirectly affected due to COVID-19 infections. The major organs that are affected are the lungs, heart, brain, kidney, liver, bladder, gastrointestinal, and reproductive organs. The field of tissue engineering can assist in repairing or regenerating the damage caused to these organs due to COVID-19 using a combination of biomaterial scaffolds, cells, and growth factors.[7] Biomaterial-based drug-delivery systems, vaccine technology, and *in vitro* model systems could be other approaches to studying disease progression and treatment.[8]

Regenerative medicine is also an important component of TERM-based approaches, comprising cell-tissue therapeutics and other cell-based products, such as exosomes, that can treat COVID-19 infections. Cell therapeutics, in this case, mainly include therapeutics based on stem cells and natural killer (NK) cells. On the other hand, exosomes act as therapeutics in the form of cell-based products.[9]

3. COVID-19 INDUCED TISSUE/ORGAN DAMAGE

Long COVID is a disease that can affect multiple organs of the body. It develops in the form of long-term effects that develop post-infection of SARS-CoV-2, and it can occur in all age groups, but it is diagnosed mostly in people between 36-50 years of age. Long COVID comprises a variety of negative consequences, with common new-onset of illnesses including myalgic encephalomyelitis/chronic fatigue syndrome (ME/CFS), postural orthostatic tachycardia syndrome (POTS), type-2 diabetes, cardiovascular, thrombotic, and cerebrovascular diseases. In situations with the development of ME/CFS and dysautonomia, symptoms can linger for years and are typically expected to last a lifetime. [10]

Immune dysfunction: One of the diseases that develop due to inflammation of the lungs and increase in permeability, leading to pulmonary oedema in acute respiratory distress syndrome (ARDS). This is due to the damage that can occur in an alveolar-capillary barrier of some COVID-19 patients leading to an acute virus-induced injury to the lung tissue. Some of the hallmarks of the hyperinflammatory phenotype of ARDS are 1) an increase in pro-inflammatory cytokine levels, 2) a higher occurrence of shock, and undesirable clinical outcomes.

The terms “cytokine storm” and “cytokine release syndrome” (CRS) are widely used interchangeably to define the dysregulation of the immune system that happens due to excessive release of cytokines leading to failure of multiple organs, systemic inflammation and increase in the death rates. CRS is characterised by the four major signs of systemic inflammatory response syndrome: fever, tachycardia, tachypnea, and hypotension. Pro-inflammatory cytokine IL-6 is one of the main modulators of the acute inflammatory response observed during ARDS and CRS. Hence, it is expected to play a role in severe symptoms associated with COVID-19 by causing hypercoagulation, hyperferritinemia, and high C-reactive protein concentrations.

In the UK, several cases of seriously ill children who had symptoms of Kawasaki disease-like systemic inflammatory response syndrome were reported. Some of these children were found to be positive for SARS-CoV-2 infection; this led to a further diagnosis of a syndrome called paediatric inflammatory, a multisystem syndrome temporally associated with SARS-CoV-2 infection (PIMS-TS), which is also known as a multisystem inflammatory syndrome in children (MIS-C). According to the reports generated through the study of over 700 cases of MIS-C (including a maximum number of cases studied in the USA alone), it was determined that this syndrome mainly occurs in children older than five years old. An additional autoimmune hypothesis was raised when one study discovered that more than 90% of COVID-19 patients tested positive for lupus anticoagulant. Since then, numerous studies have described examining COVID-19 patients for antiphospholipid (APL) antibodies.[11]

Cardiovascular damage: Initially, COVID-19 was determined primarily as an infection specific to the respiratory system. Although over time, based on various studies, it is now known to have the ability to cause infection in multiple organs. Instead of the virus directly infecting cells, the harm shown to occur across a variety of tissues is primarily linked to an immune-mediated reaction and inflammation. Endothelial dysfunction and its accompanying after-effects, including greater chances of thrombosis in deep veins, episodes of bleeding, and pulmonary embolism, indicate a disturbance in the circulatory system. Micro-clots have been observed in both cases, i.e., acute COVID-19 and delayed COVID-19, which form an important target for diagnostic and therapeutic approaches. Long-term COVID-19 has also been associated with changes in blood cell size and stiffness that may have an impact on oxygen transport.[10, 11]

Neurological and cognitive systems: Long-term COVID is associated with many neuropsychological and cognitive symptoms, such as loss of memory, the feeling of dizziness, issues related to balancing, development of sensitivity towards noise and light, cognitive damage, loss of the sense of smell and taste, *etc.* that can negatively affect the day-to-day activities of the suffering individual. Based on a survey performed on > 1.3 million people with COVID-19 infection, it was found that issues related to mental health, like anxiety and depression, slowly came back to normal. Although, the chances of developing neurocognitive conditions such as seizures, brain fog, *etc.*, were high for at least two years post-infection. [10, 11]

Reproductive system: The effect of COVID-19 on the reproductive system is often mentioned, though very few studies have been done so far to determine its pathological effect specific to each sex. In the case of women, SARS-CoV-2 infection may lead to menstrual changes in menstruating women, cause endocrine disorders, and lead to a decrease in ovarian reserves. The reason for such a response based on preliminary theories suggests that the ovarian and endometrial tissues have high numbers of ACE2 receptors. Therefore, SARS-CoV-2 can infect these tissues and disturb hormone production and endometrial response. In the case of males, both viral persistence in penile tissue and an elevated incidence of erectile dysfunction, most likely brought on by endothelial dysfunction, have been demonstrated. [10, 11]

Gastrointestinal system: Constipation, heartburn, appetite loss, nausea, and stomach discomfort are some of the long COVID gastrointestinal symptoms. Patients with COVID-19 have drastically different gut microbiota compositions called gut dysbiosis. It has been observed that people that have long COVID show a difference in the composition of gut microbiota at least until 14 months. Compared to the control groups that do not have COVID-19 infection, some microbes that show variations in the levels in COVID-19-infected individuals are elevated levels of *Ruminococcus gnavus*, *Bacteroides vulgatus*, and reduced levels of *Faecalibacterium prausnitzii*. [10, 11]

4. TERM-BASED TREATMENT STRATEGIES TO MANAGE/CURE COVID-19

This section mainly discusses the different approaches based on TERM that have so far been developed to find treatments and address the limitations of COVID-19. Some of the most commonly used treatment strategies are discussed as follows:

4.1. *Cell-based therapy*

Various cell types have been studied for COVID-19 treatment, including mesenchymal stem cells (MSCs), Natural Killer (NK) cells, early apoptotic cells, T cells, etc. As per Zaki et al., since January 2021, 89 clinical trials have been registered at *the clinicaltrials.gov* website itself. Of these, 71% comprise only clinical trials based on MSC therapy and the rest 29% of the trials are based on natural killer (NK) cells, T cells, etc.[12] Therefore, MSCs form a major impetus when it comes to cell-based therapies and the reason lies in their immunomodulatory properties along with other capabilities such as regeneration, ability to attenuate the cytokine storm generated during SARS-CoV-2 virus infection with least chances of being infected by the virus due to the lack of ACE-2 receptor which is a major entry point of the virus into human host cells, and, lastly their antimicrobial properties.[13] The trials with MSCs were conducted to study the effect after intravenous administration in COVID-19 patients, and in one such study, the alterations in immune function and the extent of inflammation were analysed, and it was observed that $ACE2^-$ MSC administration significantly improved pulmonary function and immune level.[14]

On the other hand, NK cells are a part of the innate immune system and help in viral clearance. They demonstrate therapeutic potential for the treatment of COVID-19 by helping to recognise the SARS-CoV-2 virus-infected cells and promoting the clearance of the virus. Some of the approaches which NK cells can use for therapeutic purposes in COVID-19 treatment are 1) administering immunostimulants to enhance the activity of the NK cells in COVID-19 patients; 2) recruiting drugs that are capable of blocking inhibitory receptors, e.g., NKG2A receptors of NK cells; and, 3) lastly one can use the -NK cells obtained via optimised *in vitro* culture of stem cells or genetically engineered immortalised NK cell lines.[15] The T-cell therapies that can be used for COVID-19 treatment include adoptive therapies such as recombinant cytokines, vaccine-activating T-cell therapies, using immune check-point inhibitors with/without anti-inflammatory drugs, etc.[16]

4.2. *MSC exosomes-based therapy*

Exosomes are a kind of extracellular vesicle having a diameter ≤ 200μm. Exosomes offer an attractive option for cell-free therapy, acting as drugs to alleviate disease symptoms developed due to COVID-19 infection. Some of the important and advantageous features of MSC-derived exosomes are: 1) they can evade the immune system due to lack of HLA- class I and HLA-class II antigens, 2) they can easily pass through small blood vessels due to their small size, 3) ease of storage as they do not require cryopreservatives such as DMSO (dimethyl sulfoxide) for storing that, in turn, may alter their characteristics, and, 4) since they are non-proliferative, they do not pose any risk of tumour formation due to uncontrolled cell division. These exosomes enter the cell by binding to the cell receptor and releasing their contents after merging with the cell membrane. In some cases, they can form endocytic vesicles inside the cytoplasm.[17]

Further, these exosomes can also be considered ideal candidates in drug-delivery vehicles owing to their properties, such as the possibility of off-the-shelf availability, biocompatibility, and bilipid membrane. These MSC-derived exosomes can be used for the treatment of lung pathologies that are associated with COVID-19 in the following ways: a) assist in the proliferation as well as protection of lung epithelial cells, b) assist in the reversing the inflammation of lungs, c) assist in polarising the macrophages present in the lungs, and, d) assist in reducing pulmonary oedema and permeability of lung proteins. Hence, there can be various mechanisms in which MSC-derived exosomes can assist as therapeutics in the treatment of damaged lungs and help in regaining the potential, especially in severely ill people.[18]

4.3. *In-vitro model/organoid systems*

To study any disease by mimicking a particular tissue's three-dimensional (3D) structure, three-dimensional *in vitro* models are more advantageous than two-dimensional (2D) models as a research model/tool. Therefore, 3D in vitro models form an attractive option to study the effects of COVID-19 disease on lung tissue, especially the mechanism of disease progression and the effect of various drugs/medications. This can, in turn, help find effective treatment options for curing the COVID-19 disease. Some of the examples of *in vitro* disease models that can be used for studying lung tissue pathology are the use of collagen-based hydrogels, organoids of lung tissue, fibrosis-on-chip, *etc.*[19]

Lung organoids are miniaturised 3D structures that imitate the function of lung tissue. These organoids can be made out of stem cells or lung progenitor cells that allow fast, easy and efficient testing for treating lung pathologies associated with COVID-19. These organoids can be made by methods such as liquid handling, bioprinting, 3D culture, *etc.*

Zhao *et al.* discovered evidence supporting the theory, which mentions that liver tissue damage caused in patients suffering from COVID-19 could be due to the destruction of cholangiocytes, causing an accumulation of bile acid. Therefore, such findings act as evidence for the role of organoid systems as a helpful medium to study the mechanism of the tissue damage caused by the SARS-CoV-2 virus. [20, 21] Intestine is another organ that has been studied using organoid systems for SARS-CoV-2 viral infections. The research by Lamers *et al.* shows that the culture of intestinal organoids helped in finding that enterocytes were the primary target cells acting as the site for infection of the SARS-CoV-2 virus in the intestinal tissue.[22]

4.4. *Vaccine technology & small-molecule drug delivery*

Vaccine systems based on biomaterial scaffolds or nano-particles can be promising candidates in the field of vaccine technology. Biocompatible biomaterial-based scaffolds or nano-particles act as vaccine carriers in such systems leading to targeted vaccine delivery. However, most of these vaccine technology-based systems are currently under animal trials, and efforts are required for further translation towards clinics. Another field in this direction comes from small molecule-based therapies such as monoclonal antibodies, small molecule drugs such as azithromycin and hydroxychloroquine, oligonucleotides, etc.[23, 24] Immunology research and novel delivery systems have also helped in designing vaccines that can be delivered through a mucosal route. Vaccine delivery through the mucosal route has provided strong evidence of the production of mucosa-localised IgA, such as in the lungs, which is highly beneficial. Researchers are also trying the transdermal microneedle platforms for delivering vaccines to induce a more robust immune response.[25]

5. CONCLUSIONS

COVID-19 has become the most widespread pandemic in terms of the number of people and countries affected. COVID-19 disease not only affects the lung tissue but the long-term of this disease can also be observed in many other organs such as the heart, liver, brain, *etc.* However, the direct and severe effects on the lungs make it a serious issue because that can lead to the possibility of developing ARDS. Most SARS-CoV2-affected patients gasped for oxygen because of acute damage to the lungs.

A long-term pathophysiological study is further required to determine the severe implications that may be caused due to the lung and other organ damage caused by COVID-19 disease. TERM-based strategies such as cell-based therapy, exosome-based therapy, *in vitro* model/organoid systems, and vaccine technology have indeed changed the course of medicine and how therapeutic approaches could be imagined. Out of these approaches, regenerative medicine in the form of cellular and exosome-based therapies is a promising approach based on clinical outcomes so far. The other TERM-based techniques such as *in vitro* model/organoid systems, and vaccine technology also demonstrate a considerable potential, although future explorations are required to develop commercially viable products in these areas.

ACKNOWLEDGEMENT

The authors declare no conflict of interest and acknowledge the support extended by NIIT University, Neemrana, Rajasthan, India, and MGM University, Aurangabad, Maharashtra, India, to work on the chapter. Dr Ruchi Mishra would also like to thank Dr Annasaheb S. Khemnar and Dr

Sanjay Harke at the Institute of Bioscience and Technology, MGM University, for extending their support while preparing this chapter.

REFERENCES

1. Acosta E. Global estimates of excess deaths from COVID-19. *Nature*. 2023; 613: 31-33. DoI: https://doi.org/10.1038/d41586-022-04138-w.
2. Vannini F, Mazzotti A, Stefanini N, et al. Coronavirus disease 2019 pandemic: should we delay regenerative cartilage procedures and accept the consequences, or can we find new normality? *Int Orthop.* 2020; 44(10): 2189-2190. DoI: 10.1007/s00264-020-04741-4.
3. Roseti L, Grigolo B. COVID-19 impact on musculoskeletal regenerative medicine research: maintaining lab continuity. *Int J Environ Res Public Health.* 2021; 18(11): 6110. DoI: 10.3390/ijerph18116110.
4. Broxmeyer HE, Parker GC. Impact of COVID-19 and future emerging viruses on hematopoietic cell transplantation and other cellular therapies. *Stem Cells Dev.* 2020; 29(10): 625-626. DoI: 10.1089/scd.2020.0064.
5. Szer J, Weisdorf D, Querol S, et al. The impact of COVID-19 on the provision of donor hematopoietic stem cell products worldwide: collateral damage. *Bone Marrow Transplant*. 2020; 55(10): 2043-2044. doi: 10.1038/s41409-020-0873-x.
6. Tatara AM. Role of tissue engineering in COVID-19 and future viral outbreaks. *Tissue Engg Part A.* 2020; 26(9-10): 468-474. DoI: 10.1089/ten.tea.2020.0094.
7. Aydin, A., Cebi, G., Demirtas, Z.E. et al. Combating COVID-19 with tissue engineering: a review. *Emergent Mater*. 2021; 4: 329–349. DoI: https://doi.org/10.1007/s42247-020-00138-6.
8. Shafiee A, Moradi L, Lim M, et al. Coronavirus disease 2019: a tissue engineering and regenerative medicine perspective. *Stem Cells Transl Med.* 2021; 10(1): 27-38. DoI: 10.1002/sctm.20-0197.
9. Basiri A, Pazhouhnia Z, Beheshtizadeh N, et al. Regenerative medicine in COVID-19 treatment: real opportunities and range of promises. *Stem Cell Rev Rep.* 2021; 17(1): 163-175. DoI: 10.1007/s12015-020-09994-5.
10. Ramos-Casals M, Brito-Zerón P, Mariette X. Systemic and organ-specific immune-related manifestations of COVID-19. *Nat Rev Rheumatol*. 2021; 17(6): 315-332. doi: 10.1038/s41584-021-00608-z.

11. Davis, H.E., McCorkell, L., Vogel, J.M. et al. Long COVID: major findings, mechanisms and recommendations. *Nat Rev Microbiol.* 21, 133–146 (2023). https://doi.org/10.1038/s41579-022-00846-2
12. Galipeau J, Sensébé L. Mesenchymal Stromal Cells: Clinical Challenges and Therapeutic Opportunities. *Cell Stem Cell.* 2018; 22(6): 824-833. DoI: 10.1016/j.stem.2018.05.004
13. Matthay MA. Therapeutic potential of mesenchymal stromal cells for acute respiratory distress syndrome. *Ann Am Thorac Soc*. 2015; 12 Suppl 1(Suppl 1): S54-7. DoI: 10.1513/AnnalsATS.201406-254MG.
14. Leng Z, Zhu R, Hou W, et al. Transplantation of ACE2-Mesenchymal Stem Cells Improves the Outcome of Patients with COVID-19 Pneumonia. *Ageing Dis.* 2020; 11(2): 216-228. DoI: 10.14336/AD.2020.0228.
15. Di Vito C, Calcaterra F, Coianiz N, et al. Natural killer cells in SARS-CoV-2 infection: pathophysiology and therapeutic implications. *Front Immunol.* 2022; 13: 888248. doi: 10.3389/fimmu.2022.888248.
16. Toor SM, Saleh R, Sasidharan Nair V, et al. T-cell responses and therapies against SARS-CoV-2 infection. *Immunology.* 2021; 162(1): 30-43. doi: 10.1111/imm.13262.
17. Al-Khawaga S, Abdelalim EM. Potential application of mesenchymal stem cells and their exosomes in lung injury: an emerging therapeutic option for COVID-19 patients. *Stem Cell Res Ther.* 2020; 11(1): 437. DoI: 10.1186/s13287-020-01963-6.
18. Bari E, Ferrarotti I, Saracino L, et al. Mesenchymal Stromal Cell Secretome for Severe COVID-19 Infections: Premises for the Therapeutic Use. Cells. 2020; 9(4): 924. DoI: 10.3390/cells9040924.
19. Atala A, Henn A, Lundberg M, et al. Regen med therapeutic opportunities for fighting COVID-19. *Stem Cells Transl Med.* 2021; 10(1): 5-13. DoI: 10.1002/sctm.20-0245.
20. Monteil V, Kwon H, Prado P, et al. Inhibition of SARS-CoV-2 infections in engineered human tissues using clinical-grade soluble human ACE2. *Cell.* 2020; 181: 905-913. e7
21. Zhao B, Ni C, Gao R, et al. Recapitulation of SARS-CoV-2 infection and cholangiocyte damage with human liver ductal organoids. *Protein Cell.* 2020; 11(10): 771-775. DoI: 10.1007/s13238-020-00718-6

22. Lamers MM, Beumer J, van der Vaart J, et al. SARS-CoV-2 productively infects human gut enterocytes. *Science.* 2020; 369 (6499): 50-54. DoI: 10.1126/science.abc1669.
23. Shahzamani K, Mahmoudian F, Ahangarzadeh S, et al. Vaccine design and delivery approaches for COVID-19. *Int Immunopharmacol.* 2021; 100: 108086. doi: 10.1016/j.intimp.2021.108086.
24. Lei, S., Chen, X., Wu, J. et al. Small molecules in the treatment of COVID-19. *Sig Transduct Target Ther* 2022; 7: 387. doi:10.1038/s41392-022-01249-8
25. Kumar A, Kumar A. Mucosal and transdermal vaccine delivery strategies against COVID-19. *Drug Deliv Transl Res.* 2022 May;12(5):968-972. DoI: 10.1007/s13346-021-01001-9.

CHAPTER 12

POLYMER NANOCOMPOSITES-BASED SMART INSULIN DELIVERY SYSTEM FOR DIABETES MANAGEMENT

SWAGATIKA BARIK[1],
GIRISH CHANDRA MOHANTA[2],
PRASOON KUMAR[1]

[1]Biodesign and Medical Devices Laboratory, Department of Biotechnology and Medical Engineering, NIT Rourkela, 769008, Odisha, India;
[1]Materials Science and Sensor Applications Division, CSIR-Central Scientific Instruments Organization (CSIR-CSIO), Chandigarh-160030, India

ABSTRACT

Diabetes Mellitus Type I is an autoimmune condition that prevents the pancreas from producing insulin by destroying the β-cells and resulting in hyperglycemia. Traditional methods of diabetes treatment include insulin injections, which increase the risk of infections and affect the quality of life. Alternatively, anti-diabetic drugs are prescribed, increasing insulin secretion or changing the way glucose is metabolized in the body. However, a perfect therapy that simultaneously senses blood glucose levels and adjusts insulin delivery accordingly remains elusive. In the past two decades, advances in nano and microfabrication technologies have unfurled tremendous opportunities for achieving such an intelligent insulin delivery system. Delivery systems comprising polymers or nanocomposites are at the forefront of such efforts. In this chapter, we have discussed various polymer/composite nanoparticle-based innovative insulin delivery systems. Different aspects of the delivery system, such as design, fabrication or synthesis, characterization and delivery mechanism, have been discussed.

Furthermore, various routes of administration, including oral, nasal and transdermal, as well as accompanying adaptations in the delivery system, have been deliberated. Finally, various challenges associated with developing an intelligent insulin delivery system and approaches to mitigate them, including design changes, have been discussed. The chapter will provide a comprehensive understanding of the state-of-art drug delivery systems for insulin in the management of diabetes.

Keywords: *Polymeric composite; Insulin delivery; Diabetes mellitus*

1. INTRODUCTION

Diabetes Mellitus is a fast-growing group of chronic disorders that are caused by impairment in glucose metabolism and insufficient secretion of insulin (a hormone that lowers the blood glucose level), resulting in hyperglycemia. Prolonged hyperglycemia has been linked with multiple organ damage and dysfunctions, including the retina, heart, kidney, nerves, and blood vessels. There are two major types of diabetes mellitus; Type-1 and Type-2. Type-1 diabetes mellitus is caused by insufficient insulin production due to the damaged pancreatic β-cells. Therefore, exogenous insulin is required for sustenance. On the other hand, Type-2 diabetes mellitus is caused due to insulin resistance developed in patients because of mutation in insulin receptors on the cell membrane of the islet of Langerhans cells[1,2]. Currently, about 422 million people globally are affected by diabetes, and it is expected to rise to more than half a billion by 2040 [3,4]. A sedentary lifestyle, increased levels of stress, and poor dietary habits are among the leading factors behind the increased incidences of diabetes in the younger population. According to WHO estimates, there are about 1.4 million of the youth population turn diabetic each year. Unfortunately, Diabetes Milletus cannot be reversed or cured. Therefore, prevention remains the only effective barrier against it. However, a patient can still live a normal life with routine testing, timely medicinal interventions, and certain lifestyle changes such as dietary habits and physical workouts. Diabetes mellitus is generally managed by either anti-diabetic drugs, which alter the glucose metabolism, or by exogenously administrating insulin hormone, predominantly by subcutaneous injections.

1.1 Glucose Metabolism and Diabetes

Glucose usually serves as a primary source of metabolic fuel in our body. The other macromolecules, such as carbohydrates, fats and proteins, are ultimately broken down into glucose. At the cellular level, glucose is converted to highly energetic ATP molecules, providing all the energy required to maintain life processes. Therefore, the plasma concentration of glucose is strictly regulated within a normal range (<100 mg/dL) in healthy human adults after overnight fasting [5]. There are three primary sources of plasma glucose; intestinal absorption from food, glycogenolysis, which is the breakdown of glycogen and gluconeogenesis, i.e., the production of glucose from amino acids and fats. During fasting conditions, the plasma glucose concentration depletes, which triggers its release from glycogen reserves and other metabolic sources the concentration is returned to normal. A liver hormone, glucagon, regulates this process. After a dietary intake of glucose, the plasma level rises rapidly, which triggers the release of insulin hormone from the pancreas. The insulin hormone is a dominant glucoregulatory hormone and suppresses metabolic glucose production by antagonizing glucagon and increasing glucose utilization by the liver, kidney and fat tissues. Thus, plasma glucose concentration quickly returned to normal[6]. Hence, any deficiency in the production or function of insulin can lead to hyperglycemic conditions that ultimately result in diabetes. Clinically, diabetes is diagnosed with the help of the Oral Glucose Tolerance Test (OGTT), which has been standardized by the World Health Organization (WHO). In OGTT, 75 g of glucose is fed to a person, and the plasma glucose concentration is monitored for the next 2 hours. The person is considered diabetic if the plasma glucose level is consistently higher than 200 mg/dL after 2 hours.

Alternatively, diabetes can be diagnosed if the fasting plasma glucose concentration is consistently higher than 126 mg/dL. Between 100 to 125 mg/dL, the person is considered pre-diabetic. The distinction between Type 1 and Type 2 Diabetes is also essential for its management. Type 1 diabetes is usually genetics and generally manifests in children and adolescents. The presence of auto-antibodies can clinically diagnose it. Unfortunately, it is non-reversible and requires life-long medications, including insulin therapy. Type-2 diabetes, on the other hand, is, develops over a long period due to poor lifestyle habits. The condition cannot be reversed but it can be managed by maintaining healthy lifestyle habits.

1.2 Insulin Structure

Insulin is a small globular peptide hormone released by β-cells of islets of Langerhans in the pancreas. It was first discovered in 1922 by Banting and Best while working with porcine pancreatic extracts[7]. The primary structure of insulin consists of two polypeptide chains, A and B, of 21 and

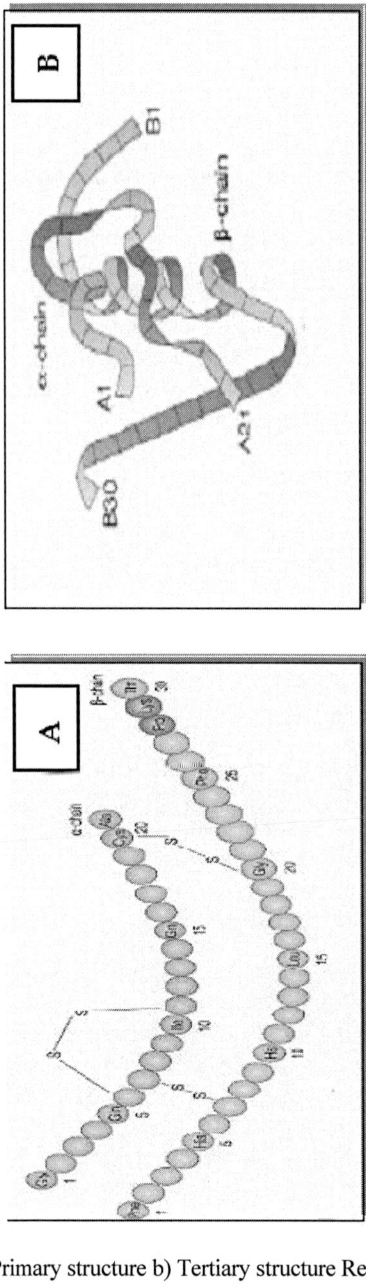

Figure 1: Insulin: a) Primary structure b) Tertiary structure Reproduced from [8], OA

30 amino acids, respectively, linked together by two disulphide bonds. The two chains are folded together in a 3D globular structure essential for insulin function. In β-cells, insulin is stored as a hexamer stabilised by zinc ions. On release into the bloodstream, it is quickly dissociated in its monomeric form, which is also the functional form of insulin. Insulin, being small in size, is rapidly transported across the body through blood circulation. On binding to cell surface receptors, insulin facilitates the translocation of glucose from plasma to the lumen of the cells through glucose transporters. Insulin primarily exerts its glucoregulatory effect in the liver, kidney, and fat tissues by promoting the synthesis of glycogen and fats. In addition, it also promotes the translocation of amino acids and potassium ions and antagonises the release of glycerol and fatty acids from adipose tissues. Thus, insulin re-balances the sudden glucose abundance by increasing its utilisation by the tissues.

1.3 Management of Diabetes Mellitus

Patients with Type 1 diabetes are unable to produce insulin naturally. Therefore, taking insulin exogenously (insulin therapy) remains the only viable option for such patients. In the case of Type 2 diabetes, insulin therapy is recommended after other alternatives for managing hyperglycemia have been exhausted. This could take 10 to 15 years after the onset of the disease. Since every individual exhibits a different glucose metabolism rate, their response to insulin therapy varies vastly.

Consequently, the insulin dosage for each individual has to be tailored by the doctors with an initial "treat-to-target" trial method[9]. This requirement for a personalised insulin dosage has emerged as a major thrust toward the development of a smart insulin drug delivery system. Such an intelligent delivery system aims to simultaneously sense the glycemic condition and regulate insulin delivery accordingly.

Insulin is a peptide hormone. Therefore, oral administration as pills is not possible, as it would destroy the hormone due to gastric juices. Therefore, direct insulin administration via subcutaneous injections was adopted as a preferred delivery route. However, there are several issues related to subcutaneous injections. For example, patients often require multiple injections of insulin throughout the day to manage their hyperglycemic condition. This often led to the development of injection phobia, particularly in young patients. Another disadvantage of multiple injections is the heightened risk of catching cutaneous infections [10]. The risk is further compounded by the fact that patients with long-term diabetes develop peripheral neuropathy and reduced blood flow. Another major threat of improper management or mistakenly taking an excess dosage of insulin therapy is the risk of hypoglycemia, which could undergo undetected or manifest into life-threatening situations [11]. Mainly, the brain and heart are at maximum risk under hypoglycemic conditions and could cause sudden death if the hypoglycemic condition is not identified and rectified soon. Other side effects include peripheral hyperinsulinemia, the development of insulin insensitivity [12], obesity due to excessive therapy [13], and eye diseases like presbyopia. Encouragingly, in the past few years, several assistive devices have been commercialised for automating insulin dosage for better management of the therapy[14].

A significant leap in the technological advancement of insulin drug delivery systems was achieved by introducing polymers as delivery vehicles for insulin [15]. The insulin activity was prolonged, and several other novel routes of administration, such as nasal, transdermal, and pulmonary, could be focused on using polymers as insulin carriers. Particularly, the coalescence of polymer science with nanotechnology brought significant improvements in insulin delivery systems[16]. Polymer nanoparticle carriers with sizes less than 100 nm can readily translocate across blood vessels, thus improving the bioavailability of insulin. Furthermore, targeted delivery of insulin can be achieved with the polymeric carrier by proper surface functionalisation with targeting moieties. This increases the bioavailability of insulin and reduces many side effects of the therapy mentioned above. Another unique advantage of polymeric carriers is that the pharmacokinetic and pharmacodynamic properties of insulin delivery systems can be easily modified by surface functionalisation. Recently, the advent of polymer composites with different nanomaterials has attracted significant research focus. These polymer nanocomposites display unique capabilities attributable to both components. For example, polymer composites with magnetic nanoparticles have been reported for magnetic-responsive insulin delivery [17]. Other polymer-based insulin delivery carriers have also been reported with responsiveness towards biological stimuli such as pH and glucose.

2. POLYMERIC NANOPARTICLES

The convergence of polymeric science with nanotechnology has created a new dimension in the field of drug delivery. Polymers are macromolecules of many repeating subunits called monomers covalently bonded to form a long linear or branched structure. The monomers can have any structure, provided they possess a minimum of two functional groups that can be linked with the functional group of another monomer to form extended structures. The distinct properties of polymers are attributed to the type of monomers used in polymerisation. Polymers can be tailored to obtain specific properties to increase a drug's bioavailability, therapeutic efficacy, and biocompatibility. These polymers also protect the drug from crossing the physical and chemical barriers and can sustain their surface charge so that they can stay in the systemic circulation, for a prolonged period, for controlled drug release at the specific site. Polymeric nanocomposites are a potential carrier for targeted/controlled drug delivery[18].

2.1 Polymeric nanomaterials as nanocarriers:

Natural polymers are obtained from natural sources. They are biocompatible and biodegradable as microorganisms can fully disassemble them and have non-toxic derivatives, which deem them suitable for insulin delivery applications. These kinds of polymers include polysaccharides like chitosan, alginate, and hyaluronic acid [19].

2.1.1 Chitosan (CS)

CS is an amino polysaccharide, made up of chitin by the deacetylation process found in the exoskeleton of crustaceans such as crabs and shrimps and in cells of the fungi harbouring β-1,4- linked N-acetyl-D-glucosamine having 1-4 glycosidic bonds [20]. It has essential properties such as biocompatibility and non-toxicity [21], acts as a coating material to protect the insulin from any proteolytic destruction [22], and has therapeutic efficacy as it helps in the prolonged release of insulin in a controlled manner [23]. Additionally, due to the N-acetyl glucosamine units, chitosan acquires a positive charge which makes it mucoadhesive. This property is harnessed to help insulin to cross through the tight junctions of the intestinal epithelial barrier, especially when administered orally [24]. However, the modified chitosan nanomaterials can be used to enhance insulin delivery by protecting it from dissolving in a few of the organic solvents and water that affects the application of the polymer in insulin delivery. It also enables the release of drugs in basic mediums and increases the therapeutic efficacy, which is the increased diffusion of drugs through the epithelial barriers, especially in the intestine. Modification like N-substitution can be performed chemically on amino groups (-NH_2), which have the functional group that is susceptible to reactions [25]. Furthermore, chitosan can form self-assembled electrostatic complexes with inversely charged macromolecules to form insulin delivery systems.

2.1.2 Alginate

Alginate, a polyanionic polysaccharide obtained from seaweed, is comprised of (1-4)-linked β-D-Mannuronopyranosyl (M) and α-L-Guluronopyranosyl (G) residues. It acts as a polyelectrolyte due to the presence of the carboxyl group and attains the property of stimuli responsiveness. Like chitosan, it has properties like biodegradability, non-toxicity, and muco-adhesiveness, making it a potential carrier for drug delivery systems. Additionally, it can react with metal ions; for example, it can restore sodium ions and set up a long chain of alginate, forming a hydrogel [26, 27].

2.1.3 Hyaluronic Acid (HA)

Hyaluronic acid, also known as hyaluronan, is a disaccharide, anionic polymer comprised of D-glucuronic acid and N-acetyl-D-glucosamine alternatively linked by β-(1-4) and β-(1-3) glycosidic bonds [26]. Due to the negative charge and stereochemistry, HA is energetically stable. Similar to chitosan and alginate, it has both the properties of biodegradability and biocompatibility and also exhibits low immunogenicity in vivo, so it is also considered a potential carrier for insulin delivery [28]. However, the modified HA and its composites, like calcium-carbonate-based composite nanocarriers with HA coatings, etc., can lead to an enhanced insulin delivery system [29], which is discussed further in this chapter.

2.2 Synthetic Polymers

Synthetic polymers are inherently hydrophobic and chemically and mechanically stronger than natural polymers. In addition, chemical resistance and mechanical robustness impart slow degradation properties to these synthetic polymers in the physiological environment. Thus, imparting high durability in any implant applications [30].

2.2.1 Poly-Lactic-co-Glycolic Acid (PLGA)

PLGA is a hydrophobic, biodegradable, biocompatible copolymer that can form a micellar structure for which it can act as a potential nanocarrier for insulin delivery. Additionally, insulin-loaded PLGA nanoparticles have the property to pass through the gastrointestinal tract by encapsulating the insulin efficiently, followed by the absorption in the walls of the intestine and releasing it in a controlled way for a longer period [31,32]. Upon ester bond hydrolysis of PLGA under physiological conditions, it breaks down into its monomeric forms, which are lactate and glycolate, followed by the release of non-toxic products from the body water and carbon dioxide. The degradation rate and the drug release kinetics of PLGA depend upon the lactic acid and glycolic acid (LA/GA) ratio and molecular weight. For instance, when the LA/GA ratio is increased, there is an increase in hydrophobicity, and a decrease in degradation and drug release rate occurs. Moreover, the degradation and drug release rates increase when the molecular weight decreases. Additionally, the amount of drug release is increased with the surface modification of the PLGA nanoparticles by PEGylation. These factors play an important role in the efficient function of PLGA nanoparticles [33, 34].

2.2.2 Poly-ε-Caprolactone (PCL)

PCL is a stable synthetic polymer with fewer ester bonds, with properties like biodegradability, biocompatibility, and controlled drug release action. Due to its fewer ester bonds, hydrolysis occurs through the action of enzymes in the body. The low degradation rates facilitate insulin delivery for a longer period. Further, its degradation product does not create an acidic environment as in the case of PGLA. It has an efficient insulin encapsulation capacity to design nanocarriers having sustained insulin delivery [31, 35].

2.2.3 Polyvinyl Alcohol (PVA)

PVA, a vinyl polymer having C-C bonds, forms a macromolecular chain. Like synthetic polymers, it has biodegradability, biocompatibility, and non-toxicity; it is also thermally stable and soluble in water [36]. However, properties can be enhanced by mixing PVA with other natural polymers to make it an efficient carrier for insulin delivery. For instance, chitosan-PVA polymers were interlinked by using glutaraldehyde for making insulin-loaded hydrogels which resulted in high permeation, considering it a potent non-invasive delivery system [37].

2.3 Stimuli-Responsive polymeric nanocarriers

The stimuli-responsive polymeric devices are responsible for the controlled release of insulin encapsulated by undergoing structural changes in response to its environmental stimuli like pH, temperature, light, enzymes, glucose, etc. These polymers should possess some important features like biocompatibility, they can load high concentrations of drugs, and show non-toxicity and non-immunogenicity to act as a potential insulin carrier system [38]. Hydrogel is a crosslinked, hydrated hydrophilic network comprising a 3D structure that can absorb a high amount of water up to 70-99% due to the presence of hydrophilic functional groups -OH, $-NH_2$, or -COOH. This is made up of various natural or synthetic polymers, and the type of polymers used in hydrogel synthesis affects the water-retaining capability. Due to the water-holding capability and the morphology, hydrogel mimics the extracellular matrix (ECM). Besides that, it is biodegradable, as it has the ability of self-degradation, and is biocompatible, as it does not trigger an immune response [39]. Furthermore, it is considered a potential insulin delivery system capable of encapsulating hydrophilic drugs like insulin [40, 41]. Moreover, the networks can be modified to prevent the inflow of external agents, which can degrade the drug enzymatically [42]. For instance, the properties like swelling, stiffness, drug release rate, and degradation essential for insulin delivery can be modified. The advantage of hydrogel is its ability to provide a controlled release of insulin in response to the concentration of blood glucose level. So, the hydrogel is considered an effective smart insulin carrier as it can change its property of swelling and permeability in response to stimuli for the controlled release of insulin [40].

3. INSULIN DELIVERY VEHICLES DESIGNED FOR ROUTES OF DELIVERY

3.1 Oral insulin delivery

Insulin delivery by the oral route is considered the most convenient and patient-friendly non-invasive technique. However, subcutaneous injections induce pain due to the current dimension of needles used in delivering insulin. Further, the site of insertion of a needle is a potent route for the spread of infection. When insulin is introduced into the systemic circulation directly, it causes complications like peripheral hyperinsulinemia, which can further lead to cancer, atherosclerosis, and others. So, to avoid such complications due to injection-based insulin delivery, oral insulin delivery can enable insulin circulation directly in the portal circulation, similar to that of a healthy, non-diabetic person. However, designing an oral insulin delivery system is quite challenging as the delivery system must allow insulin to survive the harsh acidic and enzymatic environment of the gastrointestinal tract. Further, the delivery system should facilitate permeation through the epithelial barrier of the small intestine and release insulin in portal circulation [8, 43].

The range of pH changes in the gastrointestinal tract is quite high. The pH value fluctuates from a highly acidic pH of 1.0-3.0 in the stomach to alkaline pH of 7.5 in the small intestine. A pH of 6.0-6.5 is found in the duodenum, and a pH of 7.0-7.5 in the ileum and jejunum [44]. PH-responsive polymers can utilise these pH variations for designing insulin delivery vehicles. The pH-responsive polymers have an acidic or basic group which can result in accepting or releasing protons due to the pH change in the surrounding. So, these polymers can conformationally change their structure, solubility, and swelling properties to release insulin in a controlled way at neutral pH that is in the small intestine [43].

Polymers such as chitosan and polyacrylic acid can be modified by their electrostatic charges in response to the fluctuation of pH in the surroundings due to the presence of weakly acidic or basic functional groups [45]. These types of polymers are complex with each other and are used as carrier devices for the oral delivery of insulin. For instance, chitosan/alginate nanoparticles can encapsulate the Cp1-11 peptide/insulin complexes. This Cp1-11 peptide/insulin Loaded Nanoparticle (CILN) acts as a pH-responsive system [46]. The stimuli-responsive properties of alginate and increased encapsulation rate of insulin and pH responsiveness by chitosan can be combined in a composite system to achieve a better insulin delivery system [26,47]. Due to the interaction between the carboxyl and amino groups of alginate and chitosan, respectively, the low pH causes shrinkage, gelation, and further swelling in the warmer environment of the alginate-chitosan mixture to design the chitosan/alginate core-shell structure. As a result, the chitosan/alginate nanoparticles are pH-responsive and suitable to carry insulin in the harsh acidic environment of the gastrointestinal tract [48,49].

Moreover, these chitosan/alginate nanoparticles are insoluble in water and due to the gelation, strong interaction between chitosan and alginate exists. This prevents the insulin from releasing into the gastric fluid. Therefore, compared to that of normal insulin-loaded nanoparticles, this complexed insulin with the Cp1-11 peptide (CILN) provides better bioavailability of insulin by preventing its aggregation and enabling it to be in a monomeric form. The sustained insulin release through CILN in the intestinal fluid showed a significant hypoglycemic effect [46].

In one of the studies, a pH-sensitive polyelectrolyte complex for oral insulin delivery has been developed by electrostatic attraction of two oppositely charged nanoparticles that are chitosan-coated and alginate-coated [50]. The polyelectrolyte complex provides a suitable environment for carrying the drug while showing biocompatibility, bioactive behaviour, pH sensitivity, non-toxicity, and mucoadhesiveness-like properties. It can also perform conformational changes in the change of pH [51]. Herein, self-assembly, with the oppositely charged molecules, properties of chitosan, and alginate's ability to protect the harsh environment of the gastrointestinal tract, is utilised to develop a polyelectrolyte complex [52]. Thus, these self-assembly polyelectrolyte complexes provide stable pH-sensitive systems [50].

In another system, monomethoxy polyethylene glycol- poly (lactic-co-glycolic acid) (mPEG-b-PLGA) played an important role in encapsulating insulin by acting as a matrix material. Also, it offered advantages like targeted drug delivery in a controlled way. Poly (vinyl alcohol)/ poly (hydroxypropyl methacrylate-co-methacrylic acid) can also be used as pH-sensitive semi-interpenetrating polymer network (semi-IPN) hydrogels as a potential oral insulin delivery system. Polymers with acidic groups like methacrylic acid can be used to develop pH-responsive hydrogel devices. As it can dissociate and swell in a basic medium due to the ionisation and deionisation of the acidic group, it has the capacity to release insulin at a low pH [19, 53]. The presence of a neutral, hydrophilic monomer in Hydroxypropyl methacrylate (HPMA) leads to its biocompatibility and non-toxic behaviour, making it suitable for designing drug delivery vehicles. However, it has poor swelling properties that limit its use in drug delivery applications. So, through an introduction of Poly (vinyl alcohol) (PVA), a hydrophilic linear polymer as a semi interpenetrating polymer enhances the swelling properties of the hydrogel by making double polymer networks. PVA is also introduced into the network due to its biocompatibility and good physical properties, as only pure PVA hydrogel is not stimuli-responsive [54]. So, therefore, insulin-loaded semi-interpenetrating hydrogel helps in the sustainable reduction of blood glucose levels when delivered orally by releasing insulin in response to pH [53].

Further, these insulin delivery vehicles can be tailored for targeted and efficient insulin delivery by introducing glucose-responsive components. For example, Glucose oxidase (Gox), phenylboronic acid (PBA), and glucose-binding molecules with insulin can be used as agents for the targeted delivery of insulin [55]. For instance, oral insulin delivery devices containing phenylboronic acid effectively target the overexpressed folate receptors in the intestinal epithelial cells [56]. Phenylboronic acid is used due to its stability in the physiological environment, which is low pH due to its high pKa value, making it a glucose sensor for efficient glucose-responsive insulin delivery. Hydrogels integrated with phenylboronic acid show increased swelling when exposed to high glucose concentrations. This is due to the bond's disintegration in PBA during swelling, leading to the release of insulin [55].

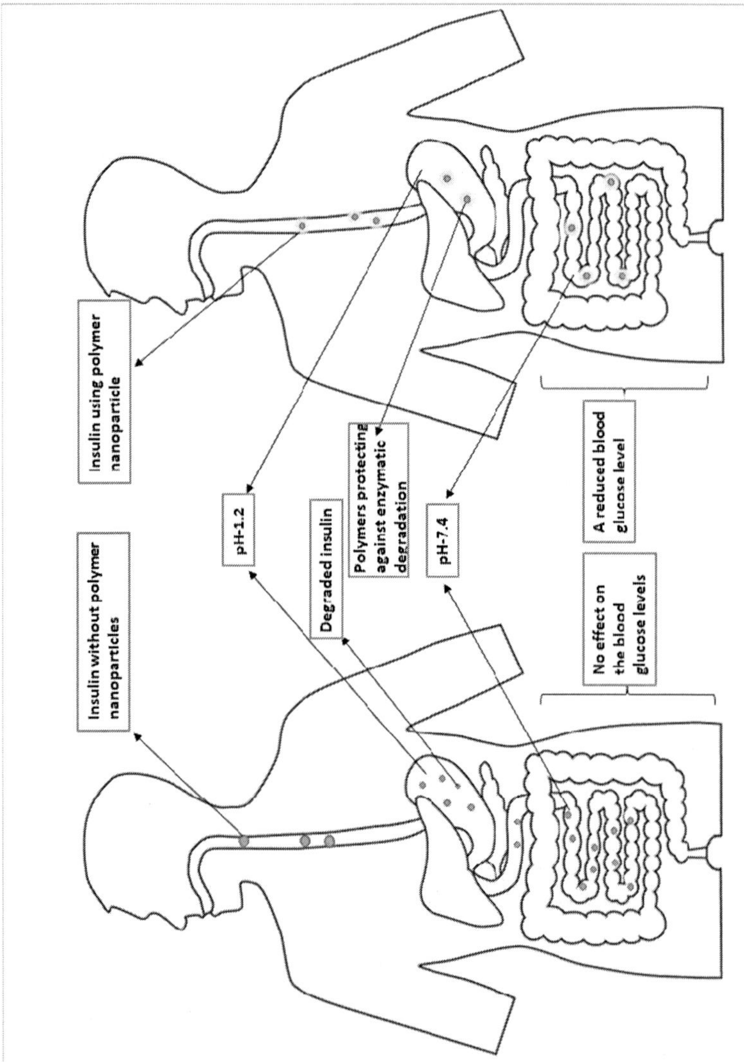

Figure 2: In vivo oral insulin delivery with and without polymeric nanoparticles

Other devices for oral insulin delivery include magnetosome-mediated delivery of insulin. Magnetosomes are intracellular, magnetite crystal structures of size 35-120nm synthesised by Magnetotactic bacteria. They have significant characteristics like narrow size distribution, which gives it a large surface area, biocompatibility, membrane-bound, non-toxicity, and paramagnetic by having a paramagnetic core of magnetite (Fe_3O_4). This crystal is covered by a magnetotactic membrane consisting of phospholipids and proteins, which also allows drugs to be encapsulated and acts as a carrier [57]. These delivery vehicles are developed by coupling method using Polyethylene glycol (PEG) to design a magnetosome-insulin complex. This coupling is achieved so that the membrane of the magnetosome having an amine group binds to the hydroxyl group in PEG, followed by insulin binding via its amine group [58]. Due to the presence of a membrane, it has the property of biocompatibility and can hold the drug due to the presence of amino acids through various conjugation techniques. Thus, making it a better carrier than the synthetically synthesised nanoparticles. Here, polyethylene glycol (PEG) is used as a crosslinking agent for the indirect coupling of magnetosome and insulin. This magnetosome complex is also protecting the insulin from the acidic environment of the gastrointestinal tract making it a favourable insulin delivery device [58,59]

3.2 Transdermal

Transdermal delivery is another alternative to painful subcutaneous injection. It can offer minimally invasive, painless delivery of insulin [60]. This route of delivery can effectively avoid the enzymatic and chemical degradation of insulin, which occurs in the oral delivery system in the gastrointestinal tract [61], and additionally, there are fewer chances of liver defects due to the first-pass metabolism [62]. Furthermore, it helps insulin to be released in a controlled fashion for a longer period. In this method, insulin has to pass the skin barrier that is the stratum corneum, the outermost skin matrix of 10-30 μm made up of lipids which do not allow large hydrophilic molecules (insulin), which act as a primary barrier. The barriers can be crossed using microneedle-based delivery systems and other systems like mechanical force-triggered and electrically facilitated strategies [61].

Microneedles are the alternative device against the subcutaneous injection of insulin administration. They are well known for their painless behaviour [61] and deliver insulin without disrupting the nerve endings while penetrating through the skin via the outermost stratum corneum and epidermis [63]. Microneedle-triggered skin punctures are temporarily created for drug transfer, and these punctures heal rapidly after removing the needle [64]. There are different kinds of microneedles according to their material and delivery processes. For example, solid microneedles puncture the skin to release the drug by the process of diffusion, and hollow microneedles, which are like normal needles but are shorter in length, allow liquid drug transfer into the layer of the skin by diffusion or injection. Furthermore, dissolving microneedles are polymeric microneedles designed from soluble biocompatible and biodegradable polymers that can help in insulin release through interaction with perspiration after responding to the glucose concentration in sweat [65].

Dissolving or biodegradable microneedles comprise soluble polymers like maltose, chitosan, and polyvinyl alcohol. The drug loading and release can be achieved through the whole needle despite coating the external surface of the needle [66]. Upon penetration of the dissolvable polymer microneedles, it gets degraded by releasing the drug loaded in it, and the by-products of the degradable polymer are non-toxic to the patient. For targeted insulin delivery through microneedles, the combination of polymers and insulin-encapsulated nanoparticles or microparticles is used to fabricate a microneedle patch device. This can provide an efficient, controlled insulin delivery, resulting in a hypoglycemic effect for an extended period [67]. The co-encapsulation of insulin and bio-responsive moieties that are glucose-responsive components of the nanoparticles are loaded into the microneedle, making it a "smart bio-responsive insulin delivery". It can deliver insulin in a specific amount in a controlled way by sensing the physiological changes when the microneedle has penetrated the skin [60]. Glucose oxidase (Gox) is the glucose-responsive moiety used to detect glucose. It is an oxidoreductase enzyme that breaks down glucose into gluconic acid by utilizing oxygen(O_2) from the body fluid to produce hydrogen peroxide (H_2O_2) when there is a high concentration of blood glucose [68]. The reaction goes as follows:

$$\textbf{Glucose+O}_2\textbf{+H}_2\textbf{O} \xrightarrow{GOx} \textbf{Gluconic acid+H}_2\textbf{O}_2 \quad \textbf{Equation 1}$$

The formation of the gluconic acid and H_2O_2 leads to a hypoxic, acidic environment that facilitates the release of insulin loaded from the microneedles and subsequently reduces the blood glucose levels by acting as hypoxia-, pH-, and H_2O_2 responsive nanoparticles [69].

3.3 Nasal

The nasal route of insulin delivery is yet another alternative route that has been explored for the non-invasive method. It is highly efficient as it bypasses the first metabolism of the liver and blood-brain barrier to facilitate the drugs directly into the systemic circulation without losing any drug due to its direct contact with the bloodstream. It is one of the favourable routes because of the large surface area of 150 cm^2 in a nasal route due to a large number of microvilli in the nasal epithelium and the high vascularity of the mucosa, which can help in drug absorption [70,71]. Despite having these advantages of nasal delivery of insulin, it has some limitations, such as low permeation and bioavailability of large molecules like insulin. Insulin cannot reside for a longer period for action in the nasal mucosa. So, various enhancers can increase the permeability and the bioavailability of larger drug molecules like insulin and increase the retention time. Many in-situ gel-forming polymers like chitosan, Poloxamer, and Carbopol are used as enhancers [43]. Poloxamers are one of the thermo- or temperature-responsive polymers composed of three polymers that are poly (ethylene oxide)-b-poly (propylene oxide)-b-poly (ethylene oxide) can be used as an in-situ gel formation system along with mucoadhesive polymers acting as a nasal formulation for insulin delivery [72,73]. Similarly, Carbopol is a supportive poly (acrylic acid) polymer for bio-adhesive drug delivery systems. It undergoes a sol-gel phase transition under the influence of pH, acting as a pH-responsive system. As a result, the insulin loaded in the gel gets released and absorbed, resulting in a hypoglycemic effect for a longer period [74,75].

Other examples of smart polymeric nanoparticles and their different delivery routes are given in Table 1.

Table 1: Examples of a few smart polymeric nanoparticles by their different delivery routes and advantages.

ROUTES	POLYMER/ COMPOSITE	SMART DELIVERY DEVICE	ADVANTAGES	REF
ORAL	Chitosan/Mucin	Chitosan-mucin complex	• Biodegradable • Biocompatible • High drug encapsulation capacity • Prolonged insulin release • Non-toxic	[76]
	Poly (ϵ-caprolactone)-Chitosan/alginate	pH-Sensitive Polymeric Poly (ϵ-caprolactone) Core-Chitosan/Alginate Shell Particle System	• Stable • pH-responsive • It shows control release of insulin • Core-shell protects insulin from the acidic environment	[35]
	Polyurethane-chitosan/alginate	Core-shell nanoparticle	• Better drug loading capacity • Controlled hypoglycemic effect • Non-toxic • Minor mucoadhesiveness	[77]
	$CaCO_3$-Hyaluronic acid	$CaCO_3$ -composite nanocarrier	• Non-toxic • Protects insulin from degradation	[29]
	Polyvinyl alcohol (PVA)/ Poly (hydroxypropyl methacrylate-co-methacrylic acid)	pH-sensitive semi-interpenetrating polymer network hydrogel	• Exceptional swelling property • Controlled pH-sensitive release of insulin	[53]

Transdermal	Hyaluronic acid, phenylboronic acid, silica	Glucose-responsive microneedle patch	• Painless • Prolonged and controlled insulin release and reduced blood glucose level	[78]
	Fluorescein isothiocyanate-poly (ethylene glycol)-covalent organic frameworks	Glucose-pH dual responsive delivery system	• Low-toxicity • Anti-diabetic effects • Biocompatible	[79]
	Carboxymethyl chitosan	Microneedle	• Increased passive diffusion • Low toxicity • Maintains weight loss	[80]
	$CaCO_3$ microparticles and poly (vinyl pyrrolidone)	Dissolving composite microneedle	• Strong mechanical strength • Remarkable swelling property • Controlled hypoglycemic effect	[67]
	Carboxymethyl cellulose	Powder carrying microneedle	• Prolonged insulin release • Deliver without fabrication loss	[81]
	Metal-organic framework (MOF)/ insulin and glucose oxidase	MOF based glucose responsive microneedle	• Can be preserved • Beneficial for emergency medical needs	[82]
Nasal	Chitosan/polyvinyl alcohol (PVA)	Thermosensitive in-situ gel system	• Reduces blood glucose levels • Shows equilibrium swelling	[83]
	Gelatin/ poloxamer	Nasal formulation	• Enhanced bioavailability • Controlled hypoglycemic effect • Reduced drug deposition in lungs	[84]
	Hydrogel-chitosan And poly (Ethylene glycol) (PEG)	Thermosensitive hydrogel-based formulation	• Controlled hypoglycemic effect for a long period of time • No toxicity • Mucoadhesive	[85]

4. FABRICATION AND CHARACTERISATION PROCESSES

The polymeric nano-delivery vehicles used for managing diabetes are stimuli-responsive and multifunctional for achieving target-specific drug delivery. For this, they have effective action in managing the disease with fewer side effects and low toxicity. So, the fabrication of this kind of polymeric nanoparticle requires more advanced nanofabrication techniques [86]. The fabrication process can be of various types for various polymers. The foremost step of developing the polymeric nanoparticle is dissolving the polymers with organic solvents to avoid toxicity-related problems.

In the emulsion-based crosslinking method, polymers like chitosan are dissolved by using an organic solvent in an oil phase to make water in oil (w/o) emulsion and then the aqueous phase is maintained by adding a surfactant (for example, polyvinyl acetate). Then, the organic emulsion is crosslinked by using a crosslinking agent (glutaraldehyde) to form precipitates, followed by the formation of nanoparticles [87]. Furthermore, core-shell nanoparticles and nanospheres are developed by the double emulsion (water/oil/water) solvent evaporation method in which the hydrophobic drug (insulin) is encapsulated. These nanoparticles facilitate drug release for a longer period with limited toxicity. They can also prevent the drug from degradation by enzymes [88]. Moreover, self-assembled insulin-loaded nanoparticles are formed by the method of sonication. In this process, there is cavitation of the drug inside the polymer, and it is a reversible process.

In recent times, microfluidics has been explored to fabricate insulin-loaded nanocomposites. A microfluidic strategy is used to fabricate the nanoparticles to speed up the mixing and enhance solvent exchange. This method can develop uniform composite nanocarriers having uniform drug distribution in the polymeric nanoparticle [86,89]. The nanoparticles can be formed by assembling natural and synthetic polymers in the microfluidic channel. For example, chitosan, hyaluronic acid, and poly (lactic-co-glycolic acid) can generate micro/nanoparticles encapsulating drugs. The microfluidic system includes the hydrodynamic flow focusing (HFF), the droplet method to micro-mix the solutions in microchannels, and the droplet method, the solvent exchange also takes place by diffusion for creating particles of uniform polydispersity index [90].

In the Sol-gel method of preparation, there is a formation of solution into a gel-like phase [91]. By this method, silica nanoparticles can be produced, encapsulating insulin. Such systems are desirable due to their small size, high surface area, and biocompatible. Here, the polymers like chitosan, alginate, and poly (ethylene glycol) can be used as a coating material to prevent the nanoparticle from degradation by the enzymes and to enhance the mucoadhesive properties of nanoparticles for easy permeability through mucous membranes [88].

The smart polymeric nanoparticles differ in their physiological properties like size, shape, loading and encapsulation efficiency, the efficiency of releasing the drug, etc. They are characterised to evaluate their drug-carrying efficiency to use those nanoparticles for effective drug delivery vehicles. For the characterisation of these nanoparticles, various methods commonly used are electron microscopy, UV-vis spectroscopy, Raman spectroscopy, Fourier Transform Infrared spectroscopy (FT-IR), chromatography, and X-ray diffraction [92,93]. For the morphological analysis, scanning electron microscopy (SEM) with XRD is used to analyse the size, shape, crystallinity, and surface structure of polymeric nanoparticles [94]. Similarly, atomic force microscopy (AFM) is used to obtain high-resolution information. For analysing the surface stiffness of these nanocarriers, AFM is being used.

The polydispersity index (PDI) determines the particle size distribution and diameter of the particles. Furthermore, to obtain information on the crystalline structure and size of the nanoparticles, the X-ray diffraction method is used [95]. The analysis of zeta potential, which is the surface charge of the polymeric nanoparticles, is important to determine the attachment of the drug to the nanoparticles [96]. Fourier Transform Infrared Spectroscopy (FT-IR) is used to determine the presence of a drug encapsulated in the nanoparticle by the presence of functional groups. In addition to that, High-performance liquid chromatography (HPLC) is used to determine the amount of drug encapsulated in the nanoparticle. Thermal analysis is carried out by differential scanning calorimetry (DSC) to determine the thermal behaviour of nanoparticles and to check the in vitro drug release. The centrifugation method analyses the amount of drug released from the nanoparticles [92, 95].

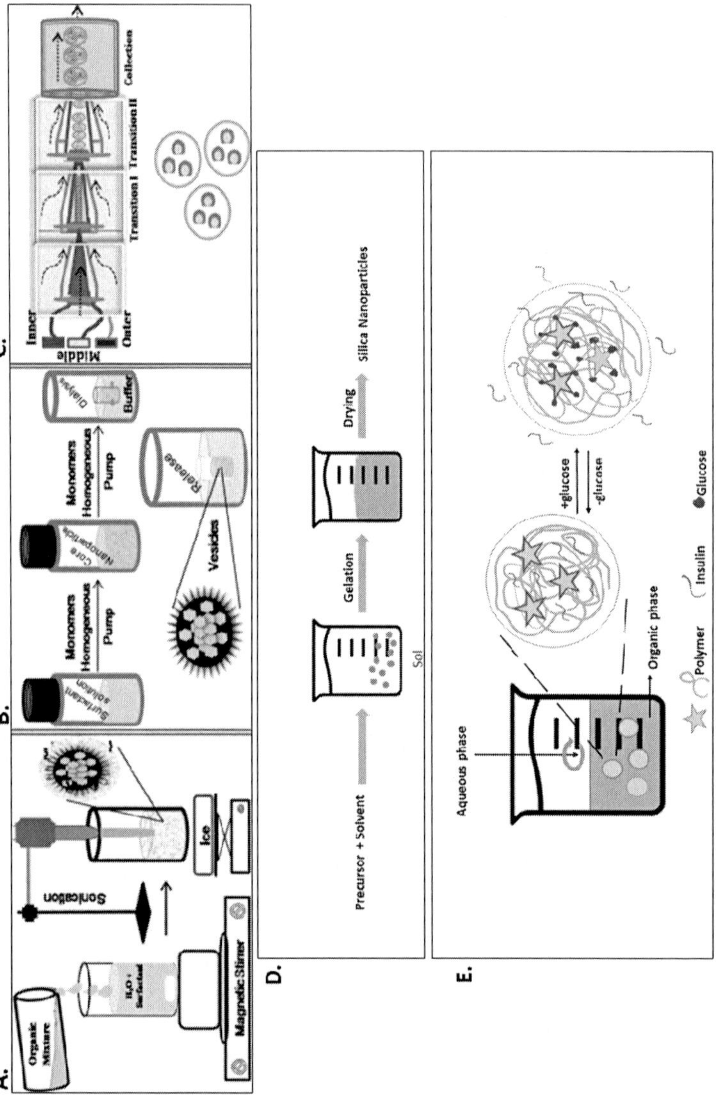

Figure 3: Fabrication Methods: A. Sonication-based method B. Core-shell particulate method C. Microfluidic method D. Sol-gel method E. Emulsion-based crosslinking method

5. MECHANISM OF ACTION

The smart insulin-loaded nanoparticles act according to the different environmental stimuli to release the drug at the targeted site. Their effect also differs according to particle size, charge, and shape.

As in oral administration, the absorption of insulin in the digestive tract depends upon the physiochemical properties of the drug, such as size, pKa (charge), solubility, and the release of the drug depends upon the suitable pH (low) of the environment. According to the size of the nanoparticles, there are various kinds of absorption mechanisms, like phagocytosis by the intestinal macrophages and endocytosis by the epithelial cells [97]. The mucoadhesive nanoparticles help in the loosening of the tight junctions and thereby increasing the uptake by transcellular and paracellular (receptor-mediated) routes [87]. When the polymeric nanoparticles are incorporated, which are cationic, they open up and release the drug-loaded nanoparticles by responding to the low pH of the intestine. Further, they interact with the anionic part of the glycoproteins in the epithelial layer of the intestine on one side and induce the change in confirmation of the F-actin on the opposite side. This results in the opening of the tight junction between the intestinal epithelial cells and allows the nanoparticles to permeate inside [98].

When the drug nanoparticles are administered in the nasal route, it comes in contact with the cilia, followed by the mucous layer. Here, the paracellular mechanism absorbs the nanoparticles, like oral insulin delivery. The nanoparticles are transported through the opening of the tight junctions present in between the nasal epithelial cell by permeation mechanism with the help of enhancers. These delivery vehicles show good bioavailability [75,99]. In the transdermal microneedle patch, when attached to the skin, the drug is released by sensing the excessive glucose by the oxidoreductase (Glucose oxidase) present in the microneedle patch. The enzyme oxidoreductase converts glucose into gluconic acid. As a result, the environments get acidic (Equation 1), followed by insulin release. The released insulin gets diffused to the stratum corneum down to the dermis migrating toward the systemic circulation achieving the target in a controlled way [100,101].

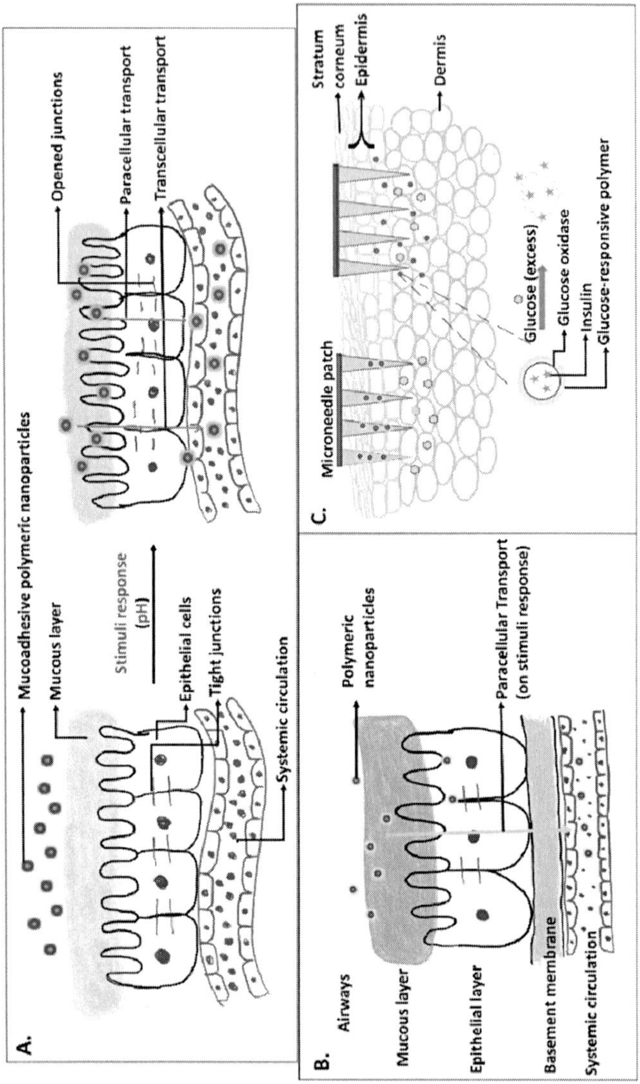

Figure 4: Mechanism of insulin-loaded polymeric nanoparticles through different routes: A. Intestinal insulin absorption through oral route B. Insulin absorption through nasal route C. Absorption through the transdermal route by microneedle

6. CHALLENGES

For insulin delivery by the smart nanoparticles, various challenges arise during the delivery of the insulin-loaded nanoparticles through different routes that are oral, transdermal, and nasal. The gastrointestinal tract is the major barrier to insulin delivery by the oral route. It is associated with the barriers like enzymes, acids, and physical barriers. The foremost challenge of the drug is to pass through the stomach containing gastric enzymes having a pH of 1.2 that can degrade the insulin, and it continues through the small intestine where the pancreatic enzymes degrade the insulin. Furthermore, when the drug reaches the small intestine, the mucous layer formed by the epithelial layer prevents the entry of the high molecular weight and large-size proteins (insulin) [21].

Similarly, in the transdermal delivery of insulin, the major challenge is the inefficient absorption of insulin due to its large molecular weight. The protective nature of the skin that prevents the passive transport of high molecular weight drugs also creates a barrier [60]. In context to the nasal insulin delivery, the drug has to pass the nasal mucosa, which is similar to the intestinal mucosa, where the drug is prevented from entering due to the tight cellular junctions [102]. Therefore, the nanoparticles should be chosen to increase the bioavailability and mucoadhesiveness of the drug formulations, and they can pass the mucous layer of the epithelial barriers efficiently and deliver the drug at the targeted site to overcome these barriers.

7. CONCLUSION

Currently, the nanocomposites-based drug delivery system is positively contributing to the field of nanomedicines. Since the discovery of insulin by recombinant DNA technology, research has been conducted to make better formulation and delivery systems to facilitate insulin delivery through different non-invasive routes. This is required as it can offer better patient compliance and mitigate stress due the invasive subcutaneous injections. The smart polymeric nanoparticle-mediated insulin delivery system has been introduced with smart stimuli-responsive polymers and is used to avoid the prolonged hypoglycemic effect by releasing the insulin in a controlled way instead of a burst release at the targeted site. Moreover, they also overcome the barriers that prevent the insulin from reaching the targeted site without causing any toxicity and reduce the complications the patients face. Thus, these smart polymeric insulin delivery systems have promising applications for the betterment of the lifestyle of diabetic patients.

ACKNOWLEDGMENTS

SB and PK thank the Science and Engineering Board (SERB), DST, Govt. of India for the financial support through a grant (SRG/2021/000859).

CONFLICT OF INTEREST

The authors declare no conflict of interest.

REFERENCES

1. Jwad SM, AL-Fatlawi HY. Types of Diabetes and Their Effect on the Immune System. Journal of Advances in Pharmacy Practices (e-ISSN: 2582-4465) [Internet]. 2022 Jun 18 [cited 2022 Sep 17];21–30. Available from: http://matjournals.co.in/index.php/JAPP/article/view/668
2. Varshosaz J. Insulin Delivery Systems for Controlling Diabetes. Recent Pat Endocr Metab Immune Drug Discov. 2008 May 14;1(1):25–40.
3. Lin X, Xu Y, Pan X, Xu J, Ding Y, Sun X, Song X, Ren Y, Shan PF. Global, regional, and national burden and trend of diabetes in 195 countries and territories: an analysis from 1990 to 2025. Scientific Reports 2020 10:1 [Internet]. 2020 Sep 8 [cited 2022 Sep 17];10(1):1–11. Available from: https://www.nature.com/articles/s41598-020-71908-9.
4. World Health Organization (WHO) [Internet]. [cited 2022 Sep 17]. Available from: https://www.who.int/
5. Giugliano D, Ceriello A, Esposito K. Glucose metabolism and hyperglycemia. Am J Clin Nutr [Internet]. 2008 Jan 1 [cited 2022 Sep 23];87(1):217S-222S. Available from: https://academic.oup.com/ajcn/article/87/1/217S/4633392.
6. Bouché C, Serdy S, Kahn CR, Goldfine AB. The Cellular Fate of Glucose and Its Relevance in Type 2 Diabetes. Endocr Rev [Internet]. 2004 Oct 1 [cited 2022 Sep 23];25(5):807–30. Available from: https://academic.oup.com/edrv/article/25/5/807/2355272.
7. BaIsU T, JouU NAL A. INSULIN. Br Med J [Internet]. 1922 Dec 12 [cited 2022 Sep 23];2(3233):1193. Available from: https://www.ncbi.nlm.nih.gov/pmc/articles/PMC2417195/

8. Elsayed AM. Oral Delivery of Insulin: Novel Approaches. Recent Advances in Novel Drug Carrier Systems [Internet]. 2012 Oct 31 [cited 2022 Sep 17]; Available from undefined/state.item.id
9. Swinnen SG, Hoekstra JB, DeVries JH. Insulin therapy for type 2 diabetes. Diabetes Care [Internet]. 2009 [cited 2022 Sep 23];32 Suppl 2(Suppl 2). Available from: https://pubmed.ncbi.nlm.nih.gov/19875560/
10. Duff M, Demidova O, Blackburn S, Shubrook J. Cutaneous manifestations of diabetes mellitus. Clin Diabetes [Internet]. 2015 Jan 1 [cited 2022 Sep 23];33(1):40–8. Available from: https://pubmed.ncbi.nlm.nih.gov/25653473/
11. McCall AL. Insulin therapy and hypoglycemia. Endocrinol Metab Clin North Am [Internet]. 2012 Mar [cited 2022 Sep 23];41(1):57–87. Available from: https://pubmed.ncbi.nlm.nih.gov/22575407/
12. Gregory JM, Cherrington AD, Moore DJ. The Peripheral Peril: Injected Insulin Induces Insulin Insensitivity in Type 1 Diabetes. Diabetes [Internet]. 2020 May 1 [cited 2022 Sep 17];69(5):837–47. Available from: https://pubmed.ncbi.nlm.nih.gov/32312900/
13. Larkin ME, Capasso VA, Chen CL, Mahoney EK, Hazard B, Cagliero E, Nathan DM. Measuring psychological insulin resistance: barriers to insulin use. Diabetes Educ [Internet]. 2008 [cited 2022 Sep 17];34(3):511–7. Available from: https://pubmed.ncbi.nlm.nih.gov/18535324/
14. Shah R, Patel M, Maahs D, Shah V. Insulin delivery methods: Past, present and future. Int J Pharm Investig [Internet]. 2016 [cited 2022 Sep 23];6(1):1. Available from: https://pubmed.ncbi.nlm.nih.gov/27014614/
15. Mansoor S, Kondiah PPD, Choonara YE, Pillay V. Polymer-Based Nanoparticle Strategies for Insulin Delivery. Polymers 2019, Vol 11, Page 1380 [Internet]. 2019 Aug 22 [cited 2022 Sep 23];11(9): 1380. Available from: https://www.mdpi.com/2073-4360/11/9/1380/htm
16. Elçioğlu HK, Sezer AD. Nanoparticle Insulin Drug Delivery — Applications and New Aspects. Application of Nanotechnology in Drug Delivery [Internet]. 2014 Jul 25 [cited 2022 Sep 23]; Available from undefined/state.item.id
17. Zhang T, Tang JZ, Fei X, Li Y, Song Y, Qian Z, Peng Q. Can nanoparticles and nano–protein interactions bring a bright future for insulin delivery? Acta Pharm Sin B. 2021 Mar 1;11(3):651–67.
18. Zielinska A, Carreiró F, Oliveira AM, Neves A, Pires B, Nagasamy Venkatesh D, Durazzo A, Lucarini M, Eder P, Silva AM, Santini A,

Souto EB. Polymeric Nanoparticles: Production, Characterization, Toxicology and Ecotoxicology. Molecules [Internet]. 2020 Aug 1 [cited 2022 Sep 17];25(16). Available from: /pmc/articles/PMC7464532/

19. Gao S, Tang G, Hua D, Xiong R, Han J, Jiang S, Zhang Q, Huang C. Stimuli-responsive bio-based polymeric systems and their applications. J Mater Chem B [Internet]. 2019 Jan 30 [cited 2022 Sep 17];7(5):709–29. Available from: https://pubs.rsc.org/en/content/articlehtml/2019/tb/c8tb02491j
20. Nayak AK, Pal DK. Chitosan-based Interpenetrating Polymeric Network Systems for Sustained Drug Release. Advanced Theranostics Materials [Internet]. 2015 Jul 17 [cited 2022 Sep 17]; 183–208. Available from: https://www.researchgate.net/publication/300173134_Chitosan-based_Interpenetrating_Polymeric_Network_Systems_for_Sustained_Drug_Release
21. Hu Q, Luo Y. Recent advances of polysaccharide-based nanoparticles for oral insulin delivery. Int J Biol Macromol. 2018 Dec 1;120:775–82.
22. Elsayed A, Al-Remawi M, Farouk A, Badwan A. Insulin-chitosan polyelectrolyte _anocomplexes: preparation, characterization and stabilization of insulin. Sudan Journal of Medical Sciences [Internet]. 2010 Aug 11 [cited 2022 Sep 17];5(2). Available from: https://www.ajol.info/index.php/sjms/article/view/57799
23. Mishra SS, Sharma A. Preparation and Characterization of Chitosan Nanoparticles of Insulin for Nasal Delivery. Journal of Drug Delivery and Therapeutics [Internet]. 2018 Oct 16 [cited 2022 Sep 17];8(5-s):400–6. Available from: http://jddtonline.info/index.php/jddt/article/view/2002
24. Tong X, Pan W, Su T, Zhang M, Dong W, Qi X. Recent advances in natural polymer-based drug delivery systems. React Funct Polym. 2020 Mar 1;148.
25. Seyam S, Nordin NA, Alfatama M. Recent Progress of Chitosan and Chitosan Derivatives-Based Nanoparticles: Pharmaceutical Perspectives of Oral Insulin Delivery. Pharmaceuticals 2020, Vol 13, Page 307 [Internet]. 2020 Oct 14 [cited 2022 Sep 17]; 13(10):307. Available from: https://www.mdpi.com/1424-8247/13/10/307/htm
26. Xie J, Li A, Li J. Advances in pH-Sensitive Polymers for Smart Insulin Delivery. Macromol Rapid Commun [Internet]. 2017 Dec 1 [cited 2022 Sep 17];38(23). Available from:

https://pubmed.ncbi.nlm.nih.gov/28976043/
27. Li M, Sun Y, Ma C, Hua Y, Zhang L, Shen J. Design and Investigation of Penetrating Mechanism of Octaarginine-Modified Alginate Nanoparticles for Improving Intestinal Insulin Delivery. J Pharm Sci [Internet]. 2021 Jan 1 [cited 2022 Sep 17];110(1):268–79. Available from: https://pubmed.ncbi.nlm.nih.gov/32663595/
28. Huang D, Chen YS, Rupenthal ID. Hyaluronic Acid Coated Albumin Nanoparticles for Targeted Peptide Delivery to the Retina. Mol Pharm [Internet]. 2017 Feb 6 [cited 2022 Sep 17];14(2):533–45. Available from: https://pubmed.ncbi.nlm.nih.gov/27997199/
29. Liu D, Jiang G, Yu W, Li L, Tong Z, Kong X, Yao J. Oral insulin delivery using CaCO3-based composite nanocarriers with hyaluronic acid coatings. Mater Lett. 2017 Feb 1;188:263–6.
30. Baghban Taraghdari Z, Imani R, Mohabatpour F. A Review on Bioengineering Approaches to Insulin Delivery: A Pharmaceutical and Engineering Perspective. Macromol Biosci [Internet]. 2019 Apr 1 [cited 2022 Sep 17];19(4):1800458. Available from: https://onlinelibrary.wiley.com/doi/full/10.1002/mabi.201800458
31. Bahman F, Greish K, Taurin S. Nanotechnology in Insulin Delivery for Management of Diabetes. Pharm Nanotechnol [Internet]. 2019 Mar 25 [cited 2022 Sep 17];7(2):113–28. Available from: https://pubmed.ncbi.nlm.nih.gov/30907328/
32. Dey GR, Saha A. Surface Engineered PLGA Nanoparticle for Threshold Responsive Glucose Monitoring and "Self-Programmed" Insulin Delivery. ACS Biomater Sci Eng [Internet]. 2021 Sep 13 [cited 2022 Sep 18];7(9):4645–58. Available from: https://pubs.acs.org/doi/full/10.1021/acsbiomaterials.1c00830
33. Rezvantalab S, Drude NI, Moraveji MK, Güvener N, Koons EK, Shi Y, Lammers T, Kiessling F. PLGA-based nanoparticles in cancer treatment. Front Pharmacol. 2018 Nov 2;9(NOV):1260.
34. Xu Y, Kim CS, Saylor DM, Koo D. Polymer degradation and drug delivery in PLGA-based drug–polymer applications: A review of experiments and theories. J Biomed Mater Res B Appl Biomater [Internet]. 2017 Aug 1 [cited 2022 Sep 17];105(6):1692–716. Available from: https://onlinelibrary.wiley.com/doi/full/10.1002/jbm.b.33648
35. Kalaycioglu GD, Elamin AA, Kinali H, Aydogan N. pH-Sensitive Polymeric Poly (ϵ-caprolactone) Core- Chitosan/Alginate Shell Particle System for Oral Insulin Delivery. ChemistrySelect [Internet]. 2021 Jan 27 [cited 2022 Sep 17];6(4):695–704. Available from:

https://onlinelibrary.wiley.com/doi/full/10.1002/slct.202004210
36. Teodorescu M, Bercea M, Morariu S. Biomaterials of Poly(vinyl alcohol) and Natural Polymers. Polymer Reviews [Internet]. 2018 Apr 3 [cited 2022 Sep 17];58(2):247–87. Available from: https://www.researchgate.net/publication/321351497_Biomaterials_of_Polyvinyl_alcohol_and_Natural_Polymers
37. Zu Y, Zhang Y, Zhao X, Shan C, Zu S, Wang K, Li Y, Ge Y. Preparation and characterization of chitosan-polyvinyl alcohol blend hydrogels for the controlled release of nano-insulin. Int J Biol Macromol [Internet]. 2012 [cited 2022 Sep 17];50(1):82–7. Available from: https://pubmed.ncbi.nlm.nih.gov/22020189/
38. Priya James H, John R, Alex A, Anoop KR. Smart polymers for the controlled delivery of drugs – a concise overview. Acta Pharm Sin B. 2014 Apr 1;4(2):120–7.
39. Mansoor S, Kondiah PPD, Choonara YE. Advanced Hydrogels for the Controlled Delivery of Insulin. Pharmaceutics 2021, Vol 13, Page 2113 [Internet]. 2021 Dec 8 [cited 2022 Sep 17];13(12):2113. Available from: https://www.mdpi.com/1999-4923/13/12/2113/htm
40. Fuchs S, Ernst AU, Wang LH, Shariati K, Wang X, Liu Q, Ma M. Hydrogels in Emerging Technologies for Type 1 Diabetes. Chem Rev [Internet]. 2021 Sep 22 [cited 2022 Sep 17];121(18):11458–526. Available from: https://pubs.acs.org/doi/full/10.1021/acs.chemrev.0c01062
41. Chen G, Tang W, Wang X, Zhao X, Chen C, Zhu Z. Applications of Hydrogels with Special Physical Properties in Biomedicine. Polymers 2019, Vol 11, Page 1420 [Internet]. 2019 Aug 29 [cited 2022 Sep 17];11(9):1420. Available from: https://www.mdpi.com/2073-4360/11/9/1420/htm
42. Li J, Mooney DJ. Designing hydrogels for controlled drug delivery. Nature Reviews Materials 2016 1:12 [Internet]. 2016 Oct 18 [cited 2022 Sep 17];1(12):1–17. Available from: https://www.nature.com/articles/natrevmats201671
43. Lin YJ, Mi FL, Lin PY, Miao YB, Huang T, Chen KH, Chen CT, Chang Y, Sung HW. Strategies for improving diabetic therapy via alternative administration routes involve stimuli-responsive insulin-delivering systems. Adv Drug Deliv Rev. 2019 Jan 15;139:71–82.
44. Evans DF, Pye G, Bramley R, Clark AG, Dyson TJ, Hardcastle JD. Measurement of gastrointestinal pH profiles in normal ambulant human subjects. Gut [Internet]. 1988 Aug 1 [cited 2022 Sep 17];29(8):1035–41. Available from: https://gut.bmj.com/content/29/8/1035

45. Mura S, Nicolas J, Couvreur P. Stimuli-responsive nanocarriers for drug delivery. Nature Materials 2013 12:11 [Internet]. 2013 Oct 23 [cited 2022 Sep 17];12(11):991–1003. Available from: https://www.nature.com/articles/nmat3776
46. Chen X, Ren Y, Feng Y, Xu X, Tan H, Li J. Cp1-11 peptide/insulin complex loaded pH-responsive nanoparticles with enhanced oral bioactivity. Int J Pharm. 2019 May 1;562:23–30.
47. Zhang J, Xia W, Liu P, Cheng Q, Tahirou T, Gu W, Li B. Chitosan Modification and Pharmaceutical/Biomedical Applications. Marine Drugs 2010, Vol 8, Pages 1962-1987 [Internet]. 2010 Jun 25 [cited 2022 Sep 17];8(7):1962–87. Available from: https://www.mdpi.com/1660-3397/8/7/1962/htm
48. Xu B, Jiang G, Yu W, Liu D, Liu Y, Kong X, Yao J. Preparation of poly(lactic-co-glycolic acid) and chitosan composite nanocarriers via electrostatic self-assembly for oral delivery of insulin. Materials Science and Engineering: C. 2017 Sep 1;78:420–8.
49. Du H, Liu M, Yang X, Zhai G. The design of pH-sensitive chitosan-based formulations for gastrointestinal delivery. Drug Discov Today. 2015 Aug 1;20(8):1004–11.
50. Chen T, Li S, Zhu W, Liang Z, Zeng Q. Self-assembly pH-sensitive chitosan/alginate coated polyelectrolyte complexes for oral insulin delivery. J Microencapsul [Internet]. 2019 Jan 2 [cited 2022 Sep 17];36(1):96–107. Available from: https://pubmed.ncbi.nlm.nih.gov/30958080/
51. Elsayed AM, Khaled AH, al Remawi MM, Qinna NA, Farsakh HA, Badwan AA. Low Molecular Weight Chitosan-Insulin Complexes Solubilized in a Mixture of Self-Assembled Labrosol and Plurol Oleaque and Their Glucose Reduction Activity in Rats. Marine Drugs 2018, Vol 16, Page 32 [Internet]. 2018 Jan 16 [cited 2022 Sep 17];16(1):32. Available from: https://www.mdpi.com/1660-3397/16/1/32/htm
52. Quiñones JP, Peniche H, Peniche C. Chitosan Based Self-Assembled Nanoparticles in Drug Delivery. Polymers 2018, Vol 10, Page 235 [Internet]. 2018 Feb 26 [cited 2022 Sep 17]; 10(3):235. Available from: https://www.mdpi.com/2073-4360/10/3/235/htm
53. Li S, Qin T, Chen T, Wang J, Zeng Q. Poly(vinyl alcohol)/poly(hydroxypropyl methacrylate-co-methacrylic acid) as pH-sensitive semi-IPN hydrogels for oral insulin delivery: preparation and characterization. Iranian Polymer Journal (English Edition) [Internet]. 2021 Apr 1 [cited 2022 Sep 17];30(4):343–53.

Available from: https://link.springer.com/article/10.1007/s13726-020-00893-7
54. Zhang Y, Song M, Diao Y, Li B, Shi L, Ran R. Preparation and properties of polyacrylamide/polyvinyl alcohol physical double network hydrogel. RSC Adv [Internet]. 2016 Nov 24 [cited 2022 Sep 17];6(113):112468–76. Available from: https://pubs.rsc.org/en/content/articlehtml/2016/ra/c6ra24006b
55. Wang J, Wang Z, Yu J, Kahkoska AR, Buse JB, Gu Z. Glucose-Responsive Insulin and Delivery Systems: Innovation and Translation. Advanced Materials [Internet]. 2020 Apr 1 [cited 2022 Sep 17];32(13):1902004. Available from: https://onlinelibrary.wiley.com/doi/full/10.1002/adma.201902004
56. Li L, Jiang G, Yu W, Liu D, Chen H, Liu Y, Huang Q, Tong Z, Yao J, Kong X. A composite hydrogel system containing glucose-responsive nanocarriers for oral delivery of insulin. Materials Science and Engineering: C. 2016 Dec 1;69:37–45.
57. Puri R, Arora V, Kabra A, Dureja H, Hamaal S. Magnetosomes: A Tool for Targeted Drug Delivery in the Management of Cancer. J Nanomater. 2022;2022.
58. Raguraman V, Jayasri MA, Suthindhiran K. Magnetosome mediated oral Insulin delivery and its possible use in diabetes management. J Mater Sci Mater Med [Internet]. 2020 Aug 1 [cited 2022 Sep 17];31(8):1–9. Available from: https://link.springer.com/article/10.1007/s10856-020-06417-2
59. Vargas G, Cypriano J, Correa T, Leão P, Bazylinski DA, Abreu F. Applications of Magnetotactic Bacteria, Magnetosomes and Magnetosome Crystals in Biotechnology and Nanotechnology: Mini-Review. Molecules [Internet]. 2018 Sep 24 [cited 2022 Sep 17];23(10). Available from: https://pubmed.ncbi.nlm.nih.gov/30249983/
60. Zhang Y, Yu J, Kahkoska AR, Wang J, Buse JB, Gu Z. Advances in transdermal insulin delivery. Adv Drug Deliv Rev. 2019 Jan 15;139:51–70.
61. Giudice EL, Campbell JD. Needle-free vaccine delivery. Adv Drug Deliv Rev. 2006 Apr 20;58(1):68–89.
62. Puoci F, Curcio M. CHAPTER 18. pH- and Temperature-responsive Hydrogels in Drug Delivery. 2013 Jun 17 [cited 2022 Sep 17];153–79. Available from: https://www.researchgate.net/publication/349466882_CHAPTER_18_pH-_and_Temperature-responsive_Hydrogels_in_Drug_Delivery

63. Xie X, Pascual C, Lieu C, Oh S, Wang J, Zou B, Xie J, Li Z, Xie J, Yeomans DC, Wu MX, Xie XS. Analgesic Microneedle Patch for Neuropathic Pain Therapy. ACS Nano [Internet]. 2017 Jan 24 [cited 2022 Sep 17];11(1):395–406. Available from: https://pubs.acs.org/doi/full/10.1021/acsnano.6b06104
64. Narayan RJ. Transdermal delivery of insulin via microneedles. J Biomed Nanotechnol [Internet]. 2014 [cited 2022 Sep 17];10(9): 2244–60. Available from: https://pubmed.ncbi.nlm.nih.gov/25992456/
65. Kwon KM, Lim SM, Choi S, Kim DH, Jin HE, Jee G, Hong KJ, Kim JY. Microneedles: quick and easy delivery methods of vaccines. Clin Exp Vaccine Res [Internet]. 2017 Jul 1 [cited 2022 Sep 17];6(2):156–9. Available from: https://doi.org/10.7774/cevr.2017.6.2.156
66. Sabri AH, Kim Y, Marlow M, Scurr DJ, Segal J, Banga AK, Kagan L, Lee JB. Intradermal and transdermal drug delivery using microneedles – Fabrication, performance evaluation and application to lymphatic delivery. Adv Drug Deliv Rev. 2020 Jan 1;153:195–215.
67. Liu D, Yu B, Jiang G, Yu W, Zhang Y, Xu B. Fabrication of composite microneedles integrated with insulin-loaded CaCO3 microparticles and PVP for transdermal delivery in diabetic rats. Materials Science and Engineering: C. 2018 Sep 1;90:180–8.
68. Zhao L, Wang L, Zhang Y, Xiao S, Bi F, Zhao J, Gai G, Ding J. Glucose Oxidase-Based Glucose-Sensitive Drug Delivery for Diabetes Treatment. Polymers 2017, Vol 9, Page 255 [Internet]. 2017 Jun 29 [cited 2022 Sep 17];9(7):255. Available from: https://www.mdpi.com/2073-4360/9/7/255/htm
69. Wang J, Zhang Y, Archibong E, Ligler FS, Gu Z. Leveraging H2O2 Levels for Biomedical Applications. Adv Biosyst [Internet]. 2017 Sep 1 [cited 2022 Sep 17];1(9):1700084. Available from: https://onlinelibrary.wiley.com/doi/full/10.1002/adbi.201700084
70. Dhuria S v., Hanson LR, Frey WH. Intranasal delivery to the central nervous system: mechanisms and experimental considerations. J Pharm Sci [Internet]. 2010 [cited 2022 Sep 17];99(4):1654–73. Available from: https://pubmed.ncbi.nlm.nih.gov/19877171/
71. Ozsoy Y, Gngör S. Nasal route: an alternative approach for antiemetic drug delivery. Expert Opin Drug Deliv [Internet]. 2011 Nov [cited 2022 Sep 17];8(11):1439–53. Available from: https://pubmed.ncbi.nlm.nih.gov/22004793/

72. Russo E, Villa C. Poloxamer Hydrogels for Biomedical Applications. Pharmaceutics 2019, Vol 11, Page 671 [Internet]. 2019 Dec 10 [cited 2022 Sep 17];11(12):671. Available from: https://www.mdpi.com/1999-4923/11/12/671/htm
73. Karavasili C, Fatouros DG. Smart materials: in situ gel-forming systems for nasal delivery. Drug Discov Today. 2016 Jan 1;21(1):157–66.
74. Nakanishi T, Kaiho F, Hayashi M. Improvement of drug release rate from carbopol 934P formulation. Chem Pharm Bull (Tokyo) [Internet]. 1998 [cited 2022 Sep 17];46(1):171–3. Available from: https://pubmed.ncbi.nlm.nih.gov/9468649/
75. Singh RM, Kumar A, Pathak K. Mucoadhesive in situ nasal gelling drug delivery systems for modulated drug delivery. Expert Opin Drug Deliv [Internet]. 2013 Jan [cited 2022 Sep 17];10(1):115–30. Available from: https://pubmed.ncbi.nlm.nih.gov/23199072/
76. Mumuni MA, Kenechukwu FC, Ofokansi KC, Attama AA, Díaz DD. Insulin-loaded mucoadhesive nanoparticles based on mucin-chitosan complexes for oral delivery and diabetes treatment. Carbohydr Polym. 2020 Feb 1;229:115506.
77. Bhattacharyya A, Nasim F, Mishra R, Bharti RP, Kundu PP. Polyurethane-incorporated chitosan/alginate core–shell nanoparticles for controlled oral insulin delivery. J Appl Polym Sci [Internet]. 2018 Jul 10 [cited 2022 Sep 18];135(26):46365. Available from: https://onlinelibrary.wiley.com/doi/full/10.1002/app.46365
78. Fu Y, Liu P, Chen M, Jin T, Wu H, Hei M, Wang C, Xu Y, Qian X, Zhu W. On-demand transdermal insulin delivery system for type 1 diabetes therapy with no hypoglycemia risks. J Colloid Interface Sci. 2022 Jan 1;605:582–91.
79. Zhang G, Ji Y, Li X, Wang X, Song M, Gou H, Gao S, Jia X. Polymer–Covalent Organic Frameworks Composites for Glucose and pH Dual-Responsive Insulin Delivery in Mice. Adv Health Mater [Internet]. 2020 Jul 1 [cited 2022 Sep 18];9(14):2000221. Available from: https://onlinelibrary.wiley.com/doi/full/10.1002/adhm.202000221
80. Zhang P, Zhang Y, Liu CG. Polymeric nanoparticles based on carboxymethyl chitosan in combination with painless microneedle therapy systems for enhancing transdermal insulin delivery. RSC Adv [Internet]. 2020 Jun 25 [cited 2022 Sep 18];10(41):24319–29. Available from: https://pubs.rsc.org/en/content/articlehtml/2020/ra/d0ra04460a

81. Kim S, Yang H, Eum J, Ma Y, Fakhraei Lahiji S, Jung H. Implantable powder-carrying microneedles for transdermal delivery of high-dose insulin with enhanced activity. Biomaterials. 2020 Feb 1;232:119733.
82. Yang XX, Feng P, Cao J, Liu W, Tang Y. Composition-Engineered Metal-Organic Framework-Based Microneedles for Glucose-Mediated Transdermal Insulin Delivery. ACS Appl Mater Interfaces [Internet]. 2020 Mar 25 [cited 2022 Sep 23];12(12):13613–21. Available from: https://pubs.acs.org/doi/full/10.1021/acsami.9b20774
83. Agrawal AK, Gupta PN, Khanna A, Sharma RK, Chandrabanshi HK, Gupta N, Patil UK, Yadav SK. Development and characterization of in situ gel system for nasal insulin delivery. Pharmazie. 2010 Mar;65(3):188–93.
84. Zhao YZ, Li X, Lu CT, Xu YY, Lv HF, Dai DD, Zhang L, Sun CZ, Yang W, Li XK, Zhao YP, Fu HX, Cai L, Lin M, Chen LJ, Zhang M. Experiment on the feasibility of using modified gelatin nanoparticles as insulin pulmonary administration system for diabetes therapy. Acta Diabetol [Internet]. 2012 Aug 29 [cited 2022 Sep 18];49(4):315–25. Available from: https://link.springer.com/article/10.1007/s00592-011-0356-z
85. Wu J, Wei W, Wang LY, Su ZG, Ma GH. A thermosensitive hydrogel based on quaternized chitosan and poly(ethylene glycol) for nasal drug delivery system. Biomaterials [Internet]. 2007 May [cited 2022 Sep 23];28(13):2220–32. Available from: https://pubmed.ncbi.nlm.nih.gov/17291582/
86. Nuxoll E. BioMEMS in drug delivery. Adv Drug Deliv Rev. 2013 Nov 15;65(11–12):1611–25.
87. Naskar S, Koutsu K, Sharma S. Chitosan-based nanoparticles as drug delivery systems: a review on two decades of research. J Drug Target [Internet]. 2019 Apr 21 [cited 2022 Sep 17];27(4):379–93. Available from: https://pubmed.ncbi.nlm.nih.gov/30103626/
88. Wong CY, Al-Salami H, Dass CR. Fabrication techniques for the preparation of orally administered insulin nanoparticles. J Drug Target [Internet]. 2021 [cited 2022 Sep 17];29(4):365–86. Available from: https://pubmed.ncbi.nlm.nih.gov/32876505/
89. Dendukuri D, Doyle PS. The Synthesis and Assembly of Polymeric Microparticles Using Microfluidics. Advanced Materials [Internet]. 2009 Nov 6 [cited 2022 Sep 17];21(41):4071–86. Available from: https://onlinelibrary.wiley.com/doi/full/10.1002/adma.200803386

90. Zhang L, Chen Q, Ma Y, Sun J. Microfluidic Methods for Fabrication and Engineering of Nanoparticle Drug Delivery Systems. ACS Appl Bio Mater [Internet]. 2020 Jan 21 [cited 2022 Sep 17];3(1):107–20. Available from: https://pubs.acs.org/doi/full/10.1021/acsabm.9b00853
91. Rane AV, Kanny K, Abitha VK, Thomas S, Thomas S. Methods for Synthesis of Nanoparticles and Fabrication of Nanocomposites. Synthesis of Inorganic Nanomaterials: Advances and Key Technologies. 2018 Jan 1;121–39.
92. Kamaraj N, Rajaguru PY, Issac P kumar, Sundaresan S. Fabrication, characterization, in vitro drug release and glucose uptake activity of 14-deoxy, 11, 12-didehydroandrographolide loaded polycaprolactone nanoparticles. Asian J Pharm Sci. 2017 Jul 1;12(4):353–62.
93. Silva AM, Alvarado HL, Abrego G, Martins-Gomes C, Garduño-Ramirez ML, García ML, Calpena AC, Souto EB. In Vitro Cytotoxicity of Oleanolic/Ursolic Acids-Loaded in PLGA Nanoparticles in Different Cell Lines. Pharmaceutics 2019, Vol 11, Page 362 [Internet]. 2019 Jul 24 [cited 2022 Sep 17];11(8):362. Available from: https://www.mdpi.com/1999-4923/11/8/362/htm
94. Bohrey S, Chourasiya V, Pandey A. Polymeric nanoparticles containing diazepam: Preparation, optimization, characterization, in-vitro drug release and release kinetic study. Nano Converg [Internet]. 2016 Dec 1 [cited 2022 Sep 17];3(1):1–7. Available from: https://nanoconvergencejournal.springeropen.com/articles/10.1186/s40580-016-0061-2
95. Sgorla D, Lechanteur A, Almeida A, Sousa F, Melo E, Bunhak É, Mainardes R, Khalil N, Cavalcanti O, Sarmento B. Development and characterization of lipid-polymeric nanoparticles for oral insulin delivery. Expert Opin Drug Deliv [Internet]. 2018 Mar 4 [cited 2022 Sep 17];15(3):213–22. Available from: https://pubmed.ncbi.nlm.nih.gov/29257904/
96. Zhang Y, Zhang L, Ban Q, Li J, Li CH, Guan YQ. Preparation and characterization of hydroxyapatite nanoparticles carrying insulin and gallic acid for insulin oral delivery. Nanomedicine. 2018 Feb 1;14(2):353–64.
97. Sharma G, Sharma AR, Nam JS, Doss GPC, Lee SS, Chakraborty C. Nanoparticle based insulin delivery system: the next generation efficient therapy for Type 1 diabetes. Journal of Nanobiotechnology

2015 13:1 [Internet]. 2015 Oct 24 [cited 2022 Sep 17];13(1):1–13. Available from: https://jnanobiotechnology.biomedcentral.com/articles/10.1186/s12951-015-0136-y

98. Artursson P, Lindmark T, Davis SS, Illum L. Effect of Chitosan on the Permeability of Monolayers of Intestinal Epithelial Cells (Caco-2). Pharmaceutical Research 1994 11:9 [Internet]. 1994 [cited 2022 Sep 17];11(9):1358–61. Available from: https://link.springer.com/article/10.1023/A:1018967116988

99. Singodia D, Kansal S, Verma A, Shukla R, Shukla P, Dwivedi P, Kumar V, Gupta P, Dwivedi AK, Mishra PR. Development of Nevirapine Loaded Novel Surfactant Free Polymeric Emulsion and Investigations for Its Suitability as Drug Delivery Vehicle. Journal of Bionanoscience. 2010 Jun;4(1–2):66–73.

100. Ye Y, Yu J, Wen D, Kahkoska AR, Gu Z. Polymeric microneedles for transdermal protein delivery. Adv Drug Deliv Rev. 2018 Mar 1;127:106–18.

101. Ahmed Saeed AL-Japairai K, Mahmood S, Hamed Almurisi S, Reddy Venugopal J, Rebhi Hilles A, Azmana M, Raman S. Current trends in polymer microneedle for transdermal drug delivery. Int J Pharm. 2020 Sep 25;587:119673.

102. Keller LA, Merkel O, Popp A. Intranasal drug delivery: opportunities and toxicologic challenges during drug development. Drug Deliv Transl Res [Internet]. 2022 Apr 1 [cited 2022 Sep 17];12(4):735–57. Available from: https://link.springer.com/article/10.1007/s13346-020-00891-5

CHAPTER 13

ESTABLISHMENT OF COMPREHENSIVE RISK ASSESSMENT PROCEDURE TO ENSURE THE SAFE OPERATION OF LHD IN UNDERGROUND HARD ROCK MINES BY INTEGRATING FRAM AND FMEA

ARVIND CHOUHAN, FALGUNI SARKAR

Department of Mining Engineering, National Institute of Technology, Rourkela (NIT-Rourkela), Rourkela, Odisha, India, Pin: 769008

ABSTRACT

The mining industry is an industry where there is a considerable amount of risk involved. Mine operators are deploying various Heavy Earth Moving Machineries (HEMM) for excavating, loading and transporting ore and waste rock/overburden. Among them, underground metalliferous mines are prime users of different HEMM having complex hydro-mechanical and auto-electric operating systems. Accidental failure in operating protocols of any such HEMM being used in underground mines can have a very distressing effect on the physical, mental and environmental health of the people involved in this industry. Besides the high compensation to be paid to the victims, an accident caused by any machines can also result in production delays which may affect the ultimate output. So, one of the essential tasks of the managers and engineers is to proactively identify the risk associated with the machines and their operating protocols and work towards minimising it. In this study, 'Functional Resonance Analysis Method' (FRAM) and 'Failure Modes and Effects Analysis' (FMEA) have been integrated to identify the hazards, assess and quantify the risks associated with the operating system of LHD (Load Haul Dumper) deployed in the underground trackless hard rock mines. Initially, the guidelines of FRAM were followed to divide the operational procedures of

LHD into different functions. Then, all the aspects of the functions were analysed by establishing a model using FRAM Model Visualizer (FMV). All the hazards associated with the identified functions had been studied by conforming to FMEA guidelines. Risk Priority Number (RPN) was calculated for all the perceived risks, and hazards were quantitatively categorised as per obtained risk levels. Risks associated with RPN greater than 150 had been addressed and negotiated urgently by taking necessary precautions. Further, numerous hazard-specific Work Plans (WP) and Standard Operating Procedures (SOP) were devised to mitigate the risks associated with the LHD operation.

Keywords: *Failure Modes and Effects Analysis (FMEA); Functional Resonance Analysis Method (FRAM); Risk Priority Number (RPN); FRAM Model Visualizer (FMV); standard operating procedure (SOP)*

1. INTRODUCTION

The mine management should understand the production needs and maintain high safety standards applicable to everyone involved to achieve success in the mining sector. The industry must identify the hazards, evaluate the related risks and continually strive to lower the risks to an acceptable level (Sarkar, 2022). The mining operations comprise significant risks to miners regarding occupational safety and health hazards. Uncertain mining circumstances and procedures produce accidents, loss and harm to human life, property damage, interruption of manufacture, etc. Risk assessment is a technique used to systematically identify and analyse the risks associated with different operations and determine the risk level of each hazard (Sarkar, Paul and Kumar, 2016). The safety of an organisation, including a mining corporation or the equipment or techniques it employs, cannot be ensured by an outside body. Therefore, the primary responsibility for ensuring safety and minimising the risks associated with the identified hazards of each specific mine unit operation is managing such a mine. In the case of the Indian mining sector, risk assessments of all machinery and activities relating to operation, maintenance, monitoring and management processes are legal requirements and governed by the DGMS (Directorate General of Mine Safety), India.

Risk assessments consist of identifying internal and external risk sources, defining the variables that may transform these risks into dangers, analysing risk priorities and determining actions to reduce risks. In various occupational health and safety management systems (e.g., OHSAS: 18001), risk evaluation is revealed as a wide-ranging method which comprises estimating the risk levels and determining the threshold limit of the risk tolerance (Ozilic, 2005). Employers should conduct a risk assessment, prepare a list of danger sources, calculate risk levels and take appropriate mitigation measures for workers' safety. The central concept in the risk assessment is to take measures to eliminate the risk source. If this is not feasible, measures should be taken to reduce the likelihood of such danger (Safe Work Australia, 2012). When risk assessment research is required to be initiated, relevant data about the work environment should be gathered. Data sources should include legislation and rules and limits, prior action and observations, statistics on accidents at work, employment statistics, employee participation, inspection reports and health and safety reports. It is essential to involve all staff in the research and seek their views while investigating (Sarkar, 2022). The primary goal of the Safety Management System is to establish proactive occupational health and safety management procedures (Sarkar, Paul and Kumar, 2016). It comprises control systems, remedial measures, feedback mechanisms, and preventative activities. Occupational health and safety (OH&S) is becoming increasingly essential in all sectors, including the environmental aspects. Safety up and downstairs has just been examined (Sandman, 2003).

In the present-day scenario, various technological changes and high-level automation in the industry have given birth to new hazards due to increment in the complexity and combination of the sophisticated processes. The operational procedures of different complex equipment can not only be controlled by technological interventions. Rather such complex control systems depend on the support and interactions with technology and human and organisational efficacy. Leveson (2004) and Rasmussen (1997) found that the failure of the components happens due to the erroneous interactions between the various systems governing the equipment's operational sequence. The Functional Resonance Analysis Method (FRAM) is extensively used to define multifaceted systems with three types of functions, i.e., technical, managerial, and human interferences. The FRAM proclaims that every function governing a system has its performance inconsistencies, and the emerging effect of these performance inconsistencies would lead to a resonance phenomenon, which may cause negative impacts on the system (Hollnagel, 2012).

FMEA was initially established in the aircraft industry in the 1960s and was utilised in the aviation sector (Australian Government, 2008). FMEA is a process for assessing possible dangers, identifying and assessing potential dangers, and proposing remedial measures to avoid risk (Bell &

Glade, 2003). FMEA is widespread in many sectors, such as aircraft, automobiles, electronics, chemicals, technology and engineering. However, few researchers have analysed hazards in mining using FMEA. Ozfirat (2013) investigated the safety condition of an underground carbon mine by using the FMEA technique. The assessment of possible dangers in underground mining through FMEA methodology and computation of Risk Priority Numbers (RPNs) had been introduced by Eyuboglu and Ozfirat (2019). Malli et al. (2017) and Balaraju et al. (2019) used FMEA in the mining industry to frame the mitigation measures for truck/dumper and machine-related accidents/incidents. They assessed possible hazards and suggested engineering measures based on early warning sensors and virtual reality solutions for the highest priorities. Shariati (2014) discovered and evaluated hazards that may arise in underground mines using FMEA. Meraj and Farhad (2015) assessed the subsidence danger in underground mines through the FMEA implementation. Oraee et al. (2011) also assessed mining risks using FMEA. The hazards associated with tunnel building through FMEA have been examined by Amini and Mojtaba (2018).

In this research, a comprehensive analysis of the operational safety of LHD operation has been conducted by integrating FRAM and FMEA. At first, the different functions and their possible inconsistencies were identified by using the FRAM methodology. The links between various functions and hazards associated with the inter-function flow paths have also been analysed. Risk levels of various hazards associated with different functions have been computed by implementing FMEA principles (Villarinho & Rodrigues, 2015). The risk of having an RPN of more than 150 was categorised as a significant hazard. Accordingly, a comprehensive, proactive risk management plan comprising work plans, Safe Operating Procedures (SOP) etc., has been designed and subjected to implementation. The judicious implementation of the methodology established in this research is expected to help the mine operators reduce the risk of LHD operation significantly.

2. DEVELOPMENT OF METHODOLOGY

As stated above, FRAM is a qualitative tool to analyse the system. It reviews the whole system by defining the functions/activities done on the system and the conditions on which each function depends. FRAM analysis of the system can be easily visualised by applying software called FRAM model visualiser. The essential postulates of FRAM analysis are:

- ➢ Establishing the goal for modelling and unfolding the condition to be analysed.
- ➢ Ascertaining the significant functions of the process, and distinguishing them, according to input, output, preconditions, resources, time, and control (as shown in Figure 1).
- ➢ Describing the actual/potential inconsistency of functions.
- ➢ Interpreting both normal and worst-case variability.
- ➢ Describing functional resonances based on potential/ actual alliances among functions.

Providing ways to monitor and minimise the inconsistency/ erraticism of performance (Hollnagel, 2012).

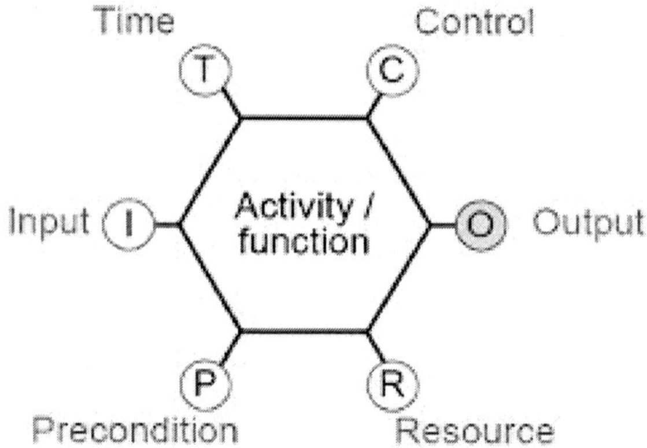

Figure 1: Various aspects of functions as per FRAM

After defining the functions and the constraints, FMEA is applied to the functions to determine the significant risks that can happen when the function/activity is carried out. FMEA is a quantitative risk assessment tool; it quantifies the risks to prioritise risks accordingly. FMEA considers three factors while calculating risks, i.e., severity (S), occurrence (O), and detectability (D).

As per FMEA methodology, the risk level is represented as RPN value which is calculated as follows:

$$RPN = S \times O \times D$$

Where S = severity, O = occurrence, and D = detectability, each ranking is based on a 10-point scale. Then, based on the value of RPN, the risk is prioritised, and action is taken. In this research, FRAM and FMEA were applied together as tools for risk management. The newly designed risk management system involves 13-step processes (as shown in Figure 2) for managing the operational hazards that evolve during the deployment of LHD in an underground hard rock mine. Implementing the designed risk management system was tested through a case study conducted in an Indian Hard Rock Mine.

3. DESCRIPTION OF MINE UNDER CASE STUDY

A declined accessed trackless underground metalliferous mine located near Tata Nagar, Jharkhand, India, was considered appropriate for the case study. The mine under investigation has implemented an overhand Cut and Fill with Post Pillar method for producing ore. The mine management has deployed jumbo drill, LHD (Load Haul Dumper) and LPDT (Low Profile Dump Truck) etc., to achieve a higher production rate and safety. The ore at stope is fragmented through the mechanised drilling and blasting system, and the transportation of fragmented rock is accomplished by LHD and LPDT combination. LHDs are versatile equipment used for conducting operations like loading, hauling and dumping. Figure 3 and Figure 4 depict the LHD equipment which is being used in the mine.

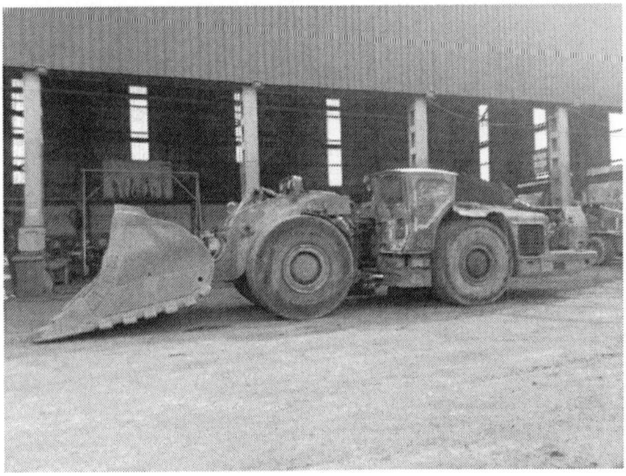

Figure 3: LHD machine at the maintenance shop

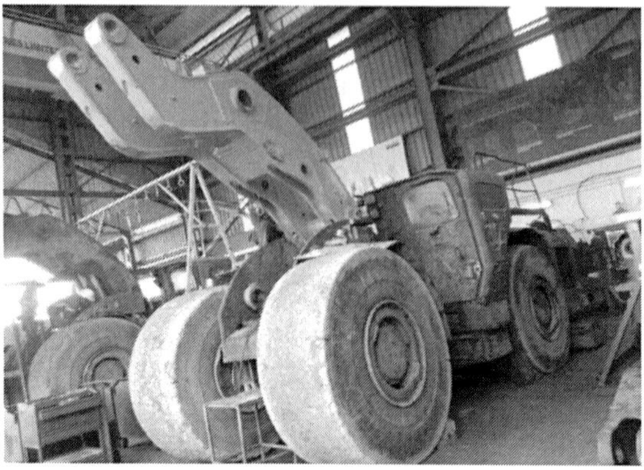

Figure 4: LHD machine during the repair.

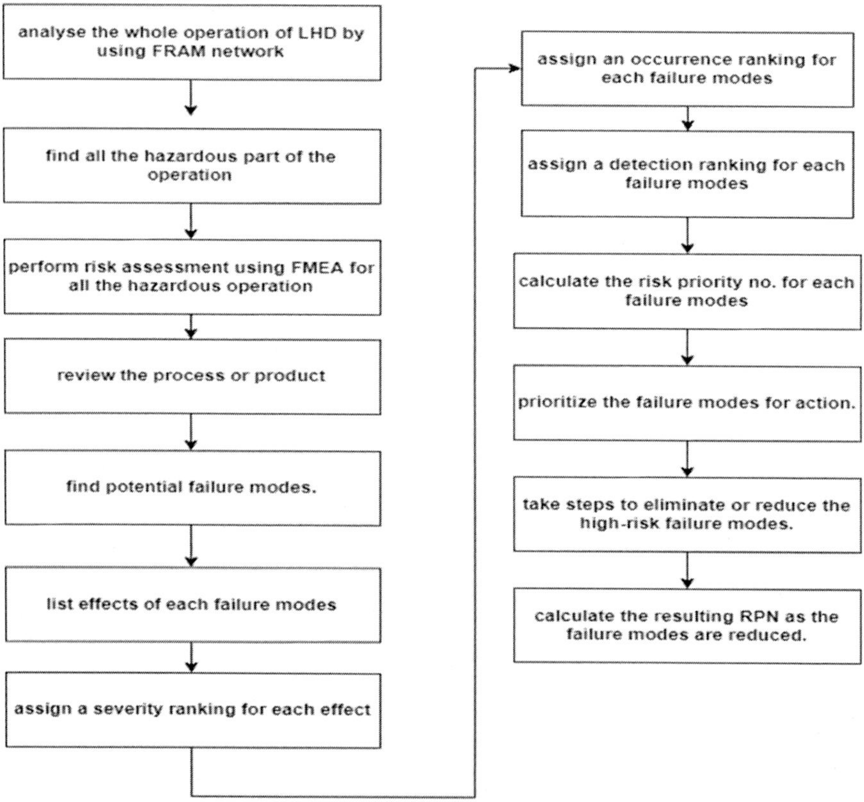

Figure 2: Development of risk management plan by integrating FRAM and FMEA

4. IMPLEMENTATION OF METHODOLOGY

First, the system-based hazard analysis on LHD is carried out using FRAM, in which we consider the processes through which LHD is deployed (from initial allocation to final mucking). Hazards associated with the recognised functional events were analysed using FMEA after consultation with the mine safety officer.

An integrated approach comprising various observations regarding LHD operation, structured interviews with the operators and maintenance crew and analysis of relevant accident statistics were adopted in this study to perform the FRAM and FMEA integration. Through FRAM analysis, essential functions governing the LHD operation were shortlisted, and hazards associated with the functions were recorded for the next study step. The functions allied with the processes had been identified along with probable variability and interactions with each other. The identified functional relations were modelled by using software called FRAM model visualiser. FMEA quantitatively analysed hazards associated with each Function. The required data for calculation of the RPN score of the hazards were generated in consultancy with the assessor team formed by the manager. Finally, risk levels of hazards were calculated, and hazards having the RPN number 150 were categorised as principal hazards. Accordingly, a hazard mitigation plan was framed and subjected to implementation

4.1. Establishment of the FRAM model

After conducting a detailed study on the recommendations of Hollnagel, 2012, observing the process of LHD operation and undergoing a brainstorming workshop involving a team of five workers from the maintenance department, eight officials and supervisors from mining, mechanical and electrical departments, three persons from LHD operators and two senior timbermen, the FRAM analysis was performed by following various steps, as discussed in the introduction section. The FRAM Model Visualizer (FMV) software was used to model the functional paths and work propagation. In the first step, different functions allied with every shift working system of LHD were identified. A function was characterised by six different features: Input (I), Output (O), Precondition (P), Resource (R), Time (T) and Control (C). An example of such analysis is shown in Table 1, considering prestart maintenance as a function of LHD operation. Detail FRAM investigation of the process is designed and depicted in **Figure 5**.

Table-1: Six aspects of FRAM functions (e.g. prestart maintenance)

Characteristic	Narrative	The instance of Function: prestart maintenance
Input(I)	That which initiates the Function	Breakdown and operation status report (previous shift)
Output(O)	The outcome of the function realisation	LHD made available for deployment
Preconditions(P)	Conditions inevitable before performing the Function	LHD is selected for deployment and has fewer operation errors and breakdown issues
Resources(R)	The material, power supply, manpower and equipment support required for the operation/ function	Maintenance crew, spare parts.
Time(T)	Time available for accomplishing the goal	Completion within 01hour from the initiation of operation/allocation
Control(C)	Management, monitoring and control	Proper supervision, choice of tools, proper PPE etc.

4.2. FMEA analysis

FMEA was applied to find the risk scores of the potential failures by giving it a value as an RPN score. First, the RPN is calculated by considering three parameters, i.e., severity (S), detection (D) and occurrence (O). The assumed values for these parameters are shown in Table 2, Table 3, and Table 4, which were assigned by **Risk Evaluation Committee** formed by the mine safety in charge. Then the RPN values are calculated for each failure, and risks are prioritised accordingly.

Table 2: Assumed values for the probability of hazard occurrence

Failure	Occurrence of failure	Degree of failure
Very high chances of failure	More than 1/2	10
	[1/3,1/2)	9
High failures	[1/8,1/3)	8
	[1/20,1/8)	7
Low	[1/80,1/20)	6
	[1/400,1/20)	5
Very low	[1/2000,1/400)	4
	[1/15000,1/2000)	3
Remote possibility	[1/150000,1/15000)	2
	Less than 1/150000	1

Table 3: Assumed values for the consequences of the occurrence of a hazard

Serial no.	Severity index	Severity description	Scale
F1	disastrous	more than four fatalities	10
F2	hazardous	one person dead or fatally injured	9
F3	extreme	more than one person severely injured	8
F4	major effect	loss of organs	7
F5	very high effect	permanent disability	6
F6	high effect	temporary disability	5
F7	moderate effect	minor fracture	4
F8	low effect	machine or component failure	3
F9	minor effect	loss in man-hour	2
F10	no effect	no effect	1

Table 4: Scale for the possibilities of hazard detection

Sl no.	Detection	Probability of detection	Detection scale
D1	absolute uncertain	0	10
D2	very remote	0.001	9
D3	remote	0.0039	8
D4	very low	0.00718	7
D5	low	0.0156	6
D6	moderate	0.062	5
D7	moderately high	0.125	4
D8	high	0.25	3
D9	very high	0.5	2
D10	almost certain	1	1

RPN is calculated using the formula RPN= S x O x D, where S = severity, O = occurrence, and D = detectability; each ranking is based on a 10-point scale. The risk categorisation system concerning RPN numbers is discussed in Table 5 below.

Table 5: Risk categorisation matrix as per FMEA

Risk class	RPN	Risk level	description
1	RPN<120	Usual	To be watched and reviewed
2	120<RPN<150	Endurable	Can be mitigated by normal safety procedures
3	RPN>150	Intolerable	Required to address immediately

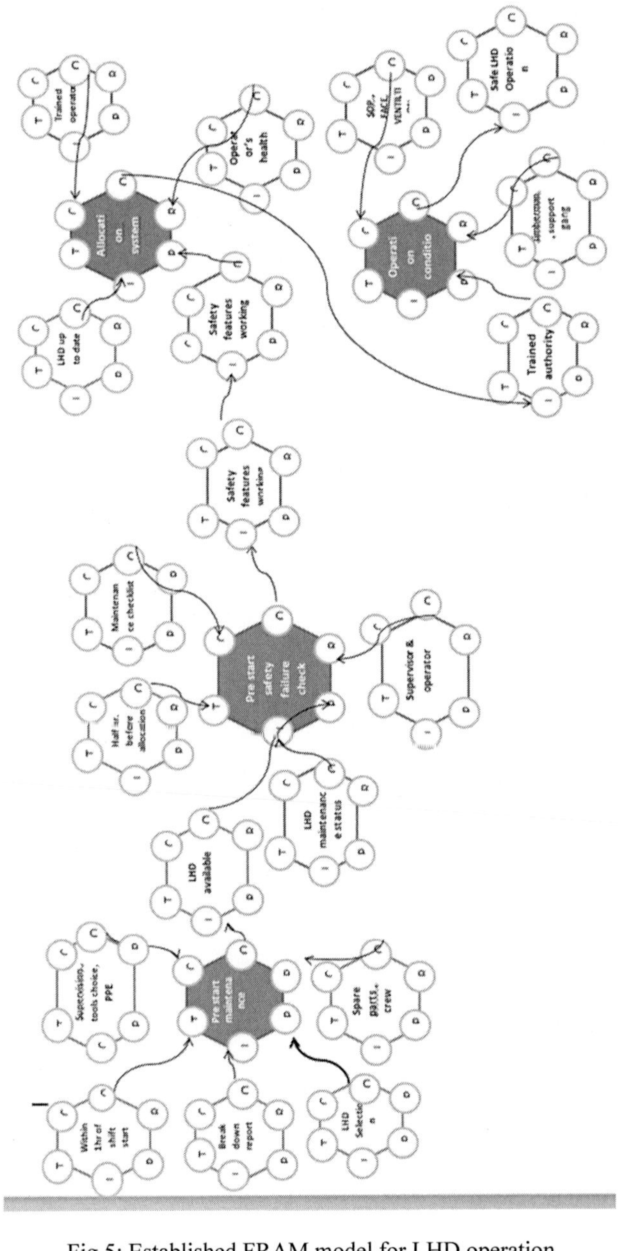

Fig 5: Established FRAM model for LHD operation

5. INTEGRATION OF FRAM AND FMEA

Here we have further analysed each Function regarding LHD operation obtained from FRAM methodology to estimate the risk associated with the functions' hazards quantitatively using the FMEA technique. Functions are shown separately in Figure 6, Figure 7, Figure 8 and Figure 9, and their aspects and assessments, along with the descriptions, are mentioned in Table 6 to Table 13.

5.1. Function 1: Prestart maintenance

Table 6: Aspects and descriptions of Function 1(Prestart maintenance)

Aspects	Descriptions
Input	Breakdown report from the previous shift
Preconditions	LHD is selected for operation
Control	Proper supervision, choice of tools, and PPE.
Time	Should be completed within 1 hr before the initiation of shift allocation
Resources	Maintenance crew, spare parts, supervisors
Output	LHD made available for deployment

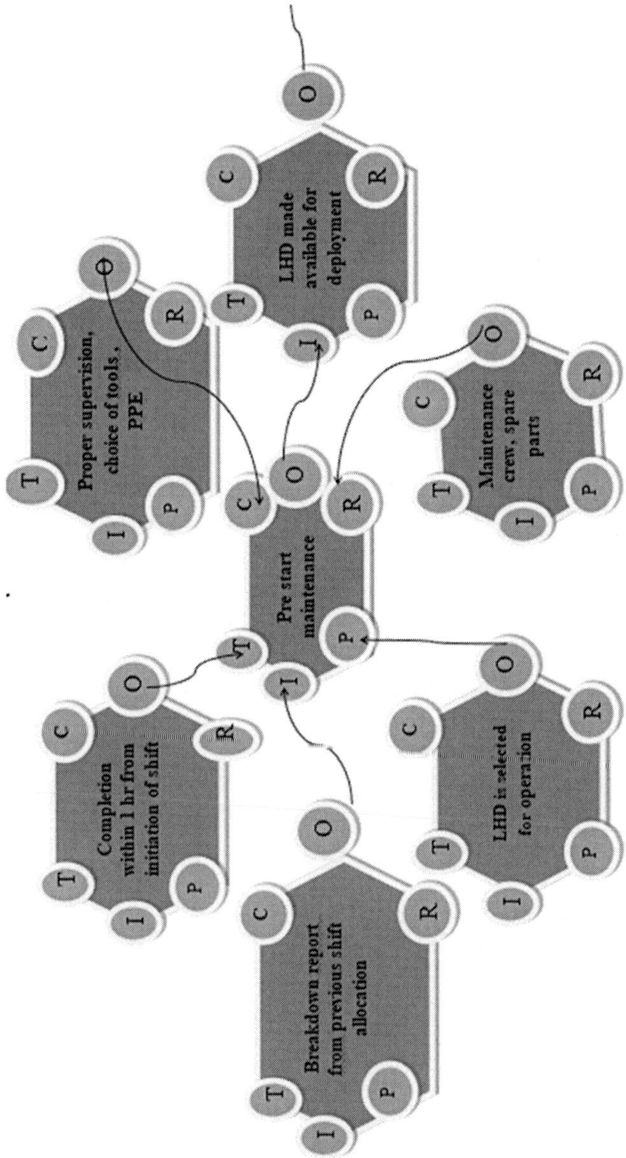

Figure 6: Function 1: Prestart maintenance

Table 7: FMEA analysis of Function 1 (Prestart maintenance)

Sl.no	Failure type	Causes	Effects	Severity	Detection	Occurrence	RPN
1	Accident while turning	Lack of focus of operator/ maintenance crew	LHD crashes with people/ object	8	5	4	**160***
2	Lack of warning sound while reversing	Defective AVA/ buzzer/ electrical system	LHD crashes with people or other machines	8	6	4	**192***
3	Lack of illumination	Inadequate Light arrangement/ electrical failure	Struck by a tool, caught in between etc	3	2	6	36
4	Tyre burst	Overpressure	Risk due to flying projectile	7	1	8	56
5	Fall on the floor due to slip	Oily garage floor	Fall on the ground	7	4	4	112
6	Heat by tools	Improper tools and lack of alertness	Hand/body part injury	2	1	4	8

* Found as significant hazards

5.2 Function 2: Prestart checks of safety features

Table 8: Aspects and description of Function 2(Prestart checks of safety features)

Aspects	Descriptions
Input	Maintenance status of LHD
Control	Maintenance checklist and operator checklist
Resources	Experienced supervisor and operator
Time	Half-hour before allocation
Precondition	LHD made available for deployment
Output	Safety features are working

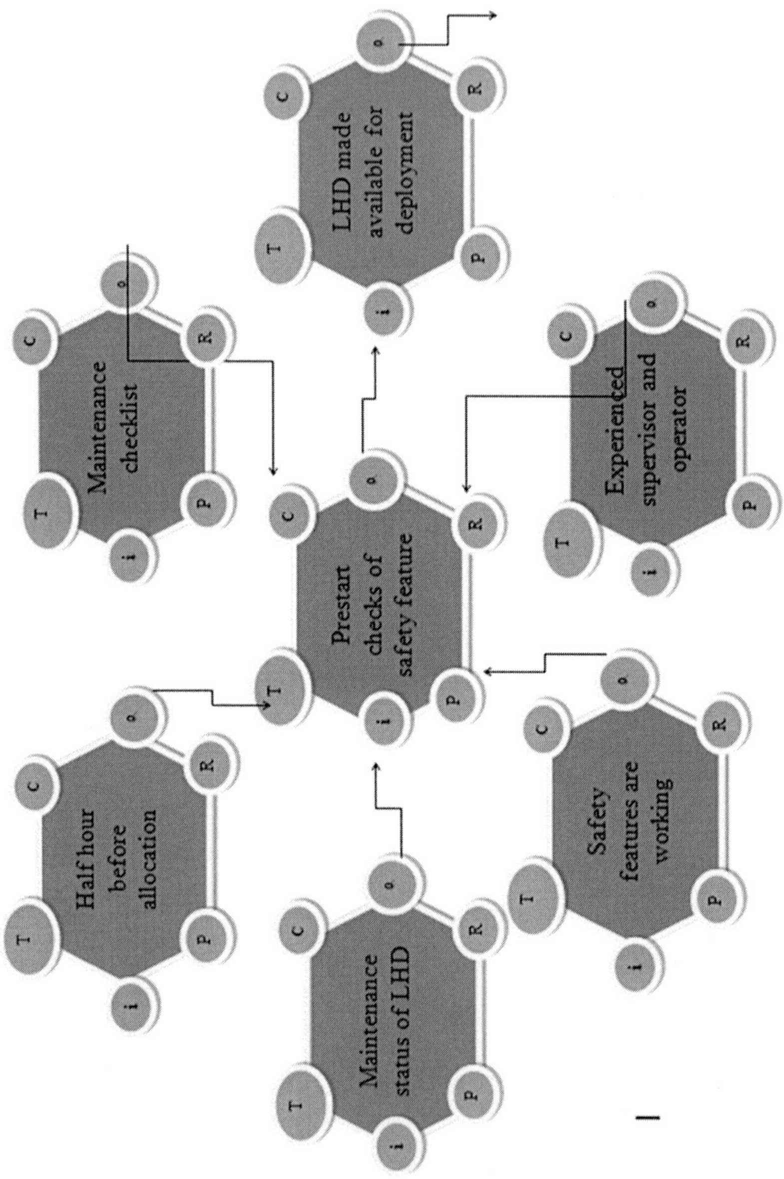

Figure 7: Function 2: FRAM analysis of LHD

Table 9: FMEA analysis of Function 2(Prestart checks of safety features)

Sl.no	Failure type	Causes	Effect	Severity	Detection	Occurrence	RPN
1	Uncontrolled LHD movement	Lack of proper maintenance	Unexpected breakdown, collision, turnover, run over	8	8	6	**384***
2	Failure in the hydraulic system	Compressor problem/ Troubleshooting avoided	Collision Brake failure, steering failure, boom failure	8	8	4	**256***
3	Failure in the braking system	Low pressure in brake oil pipe/ erosion in brake disk	Crashing on workers or object	9	3	5	135
4	Failure in the steering system	Lack of maintenance	Colliding with workers or object	4	7	6	**168***
5	Failure in the auto-electrical system	Using modified parts/non-specified parts/problem in the power circuit	Failure to start the vehicle, visibility failure,	7	3	5	105
6	Engine cooling system failure	Radiator damage	Overheating of engine/failure of engine/ Fire	8	3	6	144
7	Fuel system failure	Fuel pipe clog, fuel airlock	Complete halt of LHD	2	7	3	42

* Found as significant hazards

5.3. Function 3: Allocation System

Table 10: Aspects and description of Function no 3 (Allocation system)

Aspects	Descriptions
Input	Maintained and tested LHD
Precondition	Safety features are working
Control	Operator health condition, fatigue
Resources	An authorised and trained operator
Time	Null
Output	Allocation of trained authority

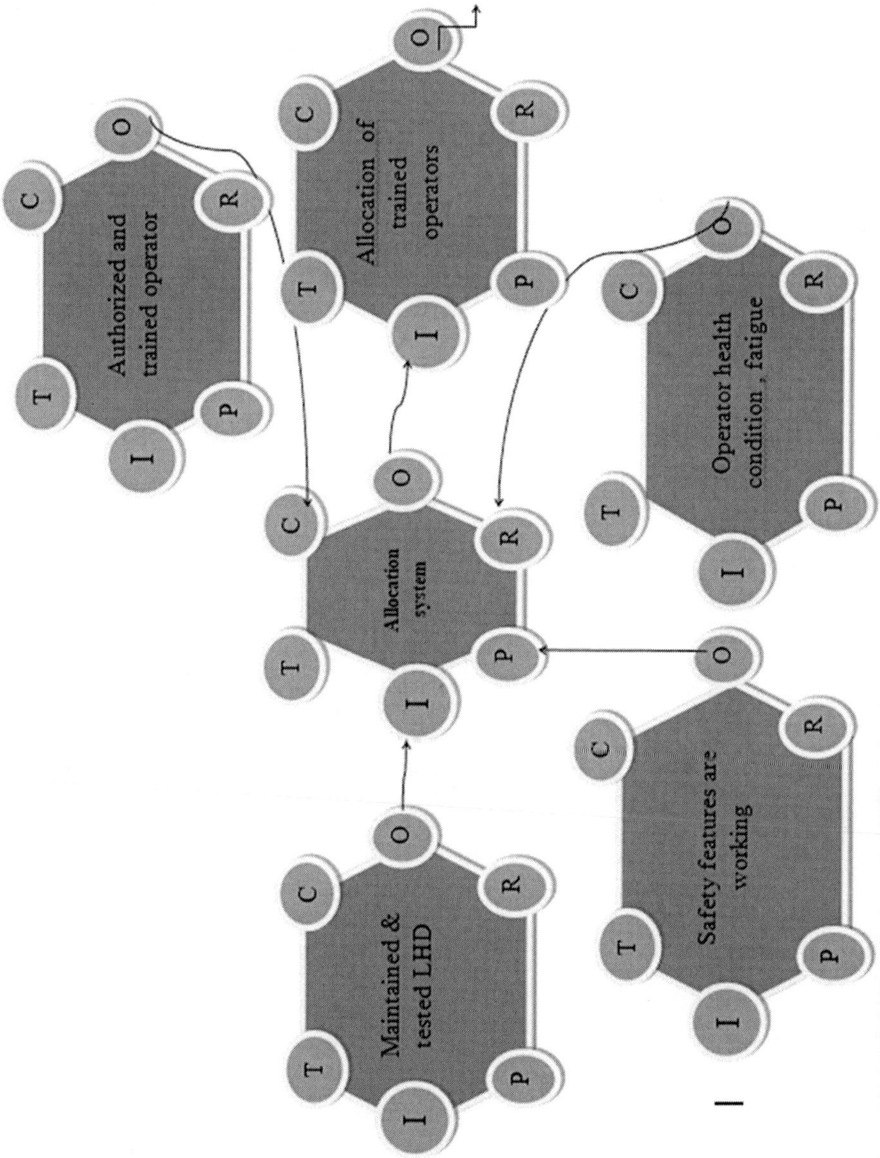

Figure 8: Function 3: Allocation system

Table 11: FMEA analysis of Function 3(Allocation system)

Sl.no	Failure type	Causes	Effect	Severity	Detection	Occurrence	RPN
1	Unskilled maintenance personnel	Maintenance protocol not followed	Unexpected breakdown during	8	8	6	**384**
2	Unskilled operator	Failure in the recruitment process	Accident due to improper handling of equipment	8	3	3	72
3	Over speeding	Operator error	Accident with people/wall	9	3	5	135
4	Unauthorised vehicle riding	Operator error	Accidents	7	6	4	**168**

* Found as significant Hazards

5.4. Function 4: Operation condition monitoring

Table 12: Aspects and Description of Function 4

Aspects	Description
Input	Properly maintained and checked LHD with the authorised operator
Resources	Timberman, support gang, supervisor
Precondition	Allocation of trained operators and supervisor
Time	Operation for a minimum 5hrs/shift
Control	SOP, face stability, ventilation, illumination, gas emission
Output	Safe LHD operation

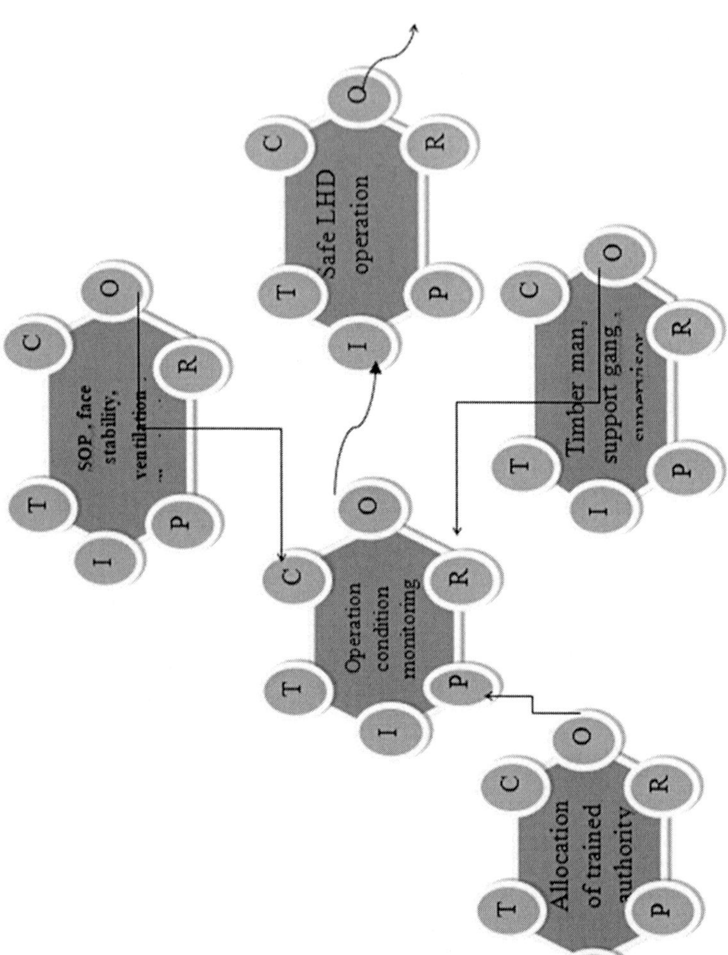

Figure 9: Function 4: Operation condition monitoring

Table 13: FMEA analysis of Function 4 (Operation condition monitoring)

Sl.no	Failure type	Causes	Effect	Severity	Detection	Occurrence	RPN
1	Lack of proper lightening	Failure of the electrical system	Crushing into people and other objects	7	4	6	**168***
2	Insufficient drift/stop width	Lack of space	Running into drift/stope wall	8	5	5	**200***
3	Lack of reflective signs at the workplace	Lack of material	Lack of visibility of walls and other structure	6	5	6	**180***
4	Blind spot	Improper camera or mirror arrangement	Risk of crushing the workers while turning or reversing	8	9	7	**504***
5	Dust	Lack of dust-suppressing system/lack of ventilation	Lack of visibility/occupational illness	7	2	5	70
6	Rock particles	Overloading of LHD/large-size rocks	Accident due to flying projectile	7	4	6	**168***
7	Improper ramp slopes	Non-maintenance of slopes	Overturning of LHD	8	6	5	**240***
8	Tyre Burst	Quality of tyre, condition of the tyre, bad haul road, over	Hit by projectile	8	4	6	**192***

Based on the integrated approach adopted, an overall hazard identification and risk assessment system for LHD operation in an underground hard rock mine has been designed. In addition, further hazard mitigation procedures in the form of work plans and Safe Operating Procedures (SOP) have been devised. Overall assessment of risks associated with various operational functions (using FRAM and FMEA) of LHD depicts that there are 14 numbers of principal hazards (shown in Table 14) allied with the system, and these hazards are required to be addressed with imperative mitigation measures. The comprehensive risk management plan comprising 42 work plans and 56 SOPs will be communicated to the mine operator for implementation. It is expected that the judicious implementation of the designed method will help mine management reduce the risk levels of identified hazards. The summary of various types of identified hazards is shown in Table 15.

Table 14: Major/Principal hazards and risk levels related to the operation of LHD in mines

Sl. No.	Failure type	Mechanism	Consequence	Severity	Detection	Occurrence	RPN
1	Accident while turning /reversing	Lack of focus of the operator	LHD crashes with people or objects	8	5	4	160
2	Lack of warning sound while reversing/turning	Defective buzzer/electrical system	LHD crashes with people or other work machines	8	6	4	192
3	The operator does not lower the moving boom and bucket when LHD is stopped	Failure in hydraulic valve/fault of the operator	Fall of moving equipment and accident risk	8	4	5	160
4	Lack of proper illumination	Light bulbs failure/electrical failure	Crushing into people and other objects/lack of visibility	7	4	6	168
5	Lack of maintenance	Too much production demand/lack of maintenance facility	Unexpected breakdown	8	8	6	384
6	Insufficient drift width	Lack of space	Running into gallery wall/overturning of LHD	8	5	5	200
7	Lack of reflective signs on haulage	Lack of material	Lack of visibility of walls and other structure	6	5	6	180

8	Blind spot	Improper camera or mirror arrangement	Risk of crushing the workers while turning or reversing	8	9	7	504
9	Dust	Lack of dust suppressing system/lack of proper ventilation	Lack of visibility/occupation al illness	7	5	7	245
10	Fly rock particles	Overloading of LHD/large-size rocks	Accident due to flying projectile	7	4	6	168
11	Improper ramp slopes	Non-maintenance of slopes	Overturning of LHD	8	6	5	240
12	Failure in the steering system	Lack of maintenance	Crashing on workers/objects	4	7	6	168
13	Unauthorised vehicle riding	Operator error	Accidents	7	6	4	168
14	Fuel system failure	Fuel pipe clog, fuel airlock	Complete halt of LHD	9	3	6	162

Table 15: Categorisation of hazards as per RPN values

Risk class	RPN	Risk level	description	No. Of hazards
1	RPN<120	Usual	To be watched and reviewed	8
2	120<RPN<150	Endurable	Can be mitigated by normal safety procedures	3
3	RPN>150	Intolerable/Principal	Required to address immediately	14

6. CONCLUSION

In this study, the researchers have examined the whole operational procedure, including conditions of workplaces associated with the operation of LHD machines in an underground hard rock mine. The qualitative assessment of the various functions allied with the operation of LHD was conducted by following FRAM postulates, and inconsistencies of all functional activities or events were analysed meticulously to identify the system-based hazards arising from the operation of LHD. After systematically reviewing the nature of the hazards, the risk levels were quantified using FMEA guidelines. The study revealed that out of 36 identified hazards, risk levels of 14 hazards have RPN values of more than 150, and they were categorised as principal or significant hazards. A total of 42 numbers of work plans have been designed and recommended for implementation to mitigate these principal hazards.

Further, comprehensive SOPs have been prepared for controlling and reducing the risk of identified hazards. The comprehensive risk assessment plan designed by integrating FRAM and FMEA methodology will be communicated to the mine operator for implementation. It is expected that the judicious implementation of the designed method will help mine management reduce the risk levels of identified hazards.

REFERENCES

1. Amini, A. and Mojtaba, F. (2018). Namaklan road tunnel risk assessment using failure mode and effect analysis (FMEA). Tunnelling and climate change conference, Tehran, Iran.
2. Australian Government, (2008). Risk assessment and management, Leading Practice Sustainable Development Program for the Mining Industry, Department of Resources Energy and Tourism, Commonwealth of Australia.
3. Balaraju, J., Govinda Raj, M., & Murthy, C. S. (2020). Prediction and assessment of LHD machine breakdowns using failure mode effect analysis (FMEA). In *Reliability, Safety and Hazard Assessment for Risk-Based Technologies: Proceedings of ICRESH 2019* (pp. 833-850). Springer Singapore.
4. Bell, R. and Glade, T., (2003). Quantitative risk analysis for landslides- Examples from Bildudalur, NW-Iceland, Natural Hazards and Earth System Sciences, 4, 117- 131.
5. Eyuboglu, K. A. and Ozfirat, M.K. (2015). Evaluating main hazards in underground metal mining by FMEA risk analysis management. Proceedings of Work Safety and Health Symposium, Adana, Turkey, 95-103.
6. F Sarkar. "Challenges Faced During the Implementation of Safety Management Plan (SMP) in Indian Underground Hard Rock Mines: A Field-Based Approach". Journal of The Institution of Engineers (India): Series D. vol.103, no.1, pp.363–373, Jan 2022.10.1007/s40033-021-00307-9
7. F. Sarkar, P.S. Paul, P. K. Prasad "An Investigation of Mine Accident/Incident Data and Implementation of Safety Management System to Minimise the Risk in a Trackless Underground Hard Rock Mine". Journal of Mines, Metals and Fuels. vol.64, no.4, pp.80-85, Apr 2016.
8. Hollnagel, E. (2017). *FRAM: the functional resonance analysis method: modelling complex socio-technical systems*. CRC Press.
9. Leveson, N. (2004). A new accident model for engineering safer systems. *Safety Science*, *42*(4), 237–270.
10. R. L. Villarinho, Assed Naked Haddad, and Paulo Victor Rodrigues de Carvalho. "Assessing risk in sustainable construction using the Functional Resonance Analysis Method (FRAM)." *Cognition, Technology & Work* 17 (2015): 559-573.
11. Malli, T. Karakus, D. Ozfirat, M. K. Gonen, A. and Kun, M. (2017). Mine truck accidents in open pit and risk assessment.

International Symposium on Occupational Health and Safety in Mining, Adana, Turkey.
12. Meraj, R. and Farhad, S.N. (2015). Prediction of subsidence risk by FMEA using artificial neural network and fuzzy inference system. International Journal of Mining Science and Technology 25: 655-663.
13. Oraee, K. Chamzini, A. and Basiri, M.H. (2011). I am evaluating underground mining hazards by fuzzy FMEA. SME Annual Meeting and Exhibit and CMA 113th National Western Mining Conference, 255-259.
14. Ozfirat, M. K. Ozfirat, P.M. Kahraman, B. Can, Y. and Oney, O. (2013). Classification of risks in the underground mine during transportation using fault mode effect analysis (FMEA). International Symposium on Occupational Health and Safety in Mining, Adana, Turkey.
15. Ozkilic, O. (2005). Occupational health and management systems and risk assessment methodologies. TISK Publishing, Ankara, Turkey.
16. Rasmussen, J. (1997). Risk management in a dynamic society: a modelling problem. *Safety Science*, *27*(2-3), 183-213.
17. Safe Work Australia (2012). Managing risks to health and safety at the workplace, fact sheet.
18. Sandman (2003). Responding to community outrage: strategies for risk management, AIHA, Fairfax, Virginia.
19. Shariati, S. (2014). An underground mine risk assessment by using FMEA in the presence of uncertainty. Decision Science Letters 3: pp. 295–304.

CHAPTER 14

NEED FOR BIOENGINEERING INNOVATIONS FOR ENVIRONMENTAL SUSTAINABILITY IN THE MINING INDUSTRY

SINGAM JAYANTHU, K. SRIDHAR REDDY, MUKTESWAR PRADHAN, PRITIRANJAN S, ANIL KUMAR INDLA

Mining Engineering Department, National Institute of Technology, Rourkela -769 008, Odisha

ABSTRACT

Bioengineering is opening up new possibilities for addressing environmental challenges. The use of genetic markers in breeding plants and animals is expanding, and bioengineered soil and genetically engineered plant species are facilitating vegetation growth in harsh environments. However, extracting natural resources through large-scale mining is necessary for the survival of the human race. Still, it can cause ecological disruption by altering land use and polluting the air, water, and soil. Mining sustainability is crucial for India to transition towards decarbonisation and meet its 2070 net-zero commitment gradually. Therefore, there is a need to implement various bioengineering techniques to establish a sustainable environmental management system in mines.

1. INTRODUCTION

Implementing long-term environmental protection measures considering social and economic factors is necessary to achieve sustainable mining practices. One such measure is the development of vegetation along mine slopes, stabilising overburdened dumps and preventing soil erosion and deterioration. Bio-engineering techniques can improve soil health and limit erosion, especially in polluted and harsh mining environments. When natural topsoil is unavailable, bio-engineered soil amendment techniques can be used to create artificial soils for land restoration. Genetically engineered plant species can be cultivated for more extended periods and in various soil types to aid in land restoration. The use of genetically modified bacteria to bioremediate soil toxicity is also being studied. As climate change and pollution threaten our future, various industries are turning to bioengineering to create sustainable and environmentally friendly solutions. Biological processes are more efficient, using less energy, water, and land than conventional methods. Bioengineering has made significant advances in producing bioplastics, biodegradable detergents, cultured meat, and low-carbon construction materials. Bioengineering can also provide sustainable alternatives to chemicals, agricultural fertilisers and harmful chemicals used to fight diseases. Biofuels derived from crops are gaining acceptance as an alternative to fossil fuels, but the competition for acreage may lead to deforestation and higher food prices. Some companies are using bacteria to transform agricultural and forestry waste into energy. Overall, the potential applications for biotechnology to promote sustainability are limitless.

2. SUSTAINABLE MINING

The mining industry in India has seen a surge in the use of advanced technology for the maximum extraction of natural resources to meet the demands of the country's growth. While this has resulted in high production rates and profits, it has come at the cost of serious ecological problems. Unfortunately, most of the technological innovations in the manufacturing process have been made without considering the impact on the environment or ecology. This has resulted in the loss of prime agricultural land, forest cover, water regime, and biodiversity.

As global environmental consciousness grew, the concept of sustainability gained favour, and the mining industry in India realised the need for sustained development. Despite enormous challenges, the mineral and mining business has the potential for sustained development. Almost every industry today offers investment opportunities that foster technological growth, exploration, mining, mineral beneficiation, mining equipment, mineral usage, and environmental protection.

Sustainable development is the biggest challenge facing human society in the 21st century. Our primary concern should be to minimise environmental disruption while sustaining economic growth and quality of life. The mining sector has increasingly adopted sustainable development principles over time. The Ministry of Coal in India is ensuring enough coal is available to meet the rising demand for energy from various industries while also prioritising care for the local environment and host community.

The coal industry is advancing a sustainable development model in which coal generation coexists with actions to conserve the environment, forests, and biological variety. The Ministry of Coal established the Sustainable Development Cell (SDC) in December 2019 to promote environmentally sustainable coal mining in the country and resolve environmental issues during mining operations until the decommissioning or complete closure of mines.

Since new private companies will play a significant role in the future coal supply matrix, the SDC's role becomes even more critical. The SDC offers recommendations, guidance, plans, and oversight for the mitigation measures taken by coal companies to maximise the sustainable use of resources, lessen the adverse effects of mining, and mitigate additional ecosystem services.

One of the focus areas of the SDC is land improvement and afforestation, which explores the functional integration of modern reclaimed land. The SDC employs a comprehensive strategy that includes gathering and analysing data, planning by subject matter experts, implementing best practices, consulting with stakeholders, creative thinking, site-specific approaches, and disseminating the results. SDC aims to enhance the quality of life for people and communities living in and around mining areas.

In summary, the Indian mining industry has made significant strides in adopting sustainable development principles, recognising the importance of coexisting with the environment while meeting the demands for natural resources. Establishing the Sustainable Development Cell is a promising initiative that will drive environmentally sustainable coal mining in India and ensure the long-term viability of the coal sector.

3. BIOLOGICAL MINE RECLAMATION AS A SUSTAINABILITY INDICATOR

Reclaiming degraded land through biological means with a specific end-use in mind is an environmentally sustainable option that has the potential to mitigate the negative impacts of mining. When restoring abandoned mineral sites, one of the primary challenges is establishing and maintaining vegetation on disturbed land. This is because mining activities can severely impact soil's chemical and physical characteristics, making it difficult for vegetation to grow. One of the most common problems with mining waste is the lack of topsoil, which is vital for plant growth. Nitrogen, another essential component of plant growth, is also often scarce in mining waste. This is due to the lack of soil organic matter, which is usually produced by decomposing dead plant matter. In addition, the decomposition of plant debris is hindered by the absence of soil microorganisms. On top of this, mine waste is typically stony and retains water, making it difficult for vegetation to grow and water to infiltrate the soil.

Selective planting of appropriate native species is often preferred over allowing natural vegetation to take its course to overcome these challenges. This is because the natural vegetation process on mine waste can be extremely slow, and mining engineers may prefer to simply plant some species on the barren land. However, to establish a permanent vegetation cover, developing a plant community that can sustain itself without human intervention is important. Various environmental factors need to be considered when selecting species for a plantation to achieve this. This includes enhancing the organic content and accessible nutrients in the soil, stabilising the soil, and encouraging the growth of understories.

It is recommended to plant quick-growing grasses with short life cycles and legumes and fodder crops in the early stages to promote successful vegetation. This helps to increase the amount of organic matter and nutrients in the soil. Over time, planting mixed species can help to further restore the ecosystem. It is important to note that restoring abandoned land with self-sustaining vegetation can help to restore the productivity of the land and the natural capital of flora and wildlife that may have been impacted by mining activities. Ultimately, successful biological reclamation can help to mitigate the negative impacts of mining and promote environmental sustainability.

4. BIOREMEDIATION OF MINED-OUT SOIL

Restoring degraded mine overburden (OB) or abandoned mining sites is a major environmental challenge. The characteristics of mining OB are not conducive to plant growth, as it lacks true soil characteristics and contains no macro- and micronutrients. In addition, it is often contaminated with trace and heavy metals. A viable approach to restoring the mine waste dumps is to plant a mix of herbaceous plants, shrubs, cover crops, and tree species for 3 to 5 years to promote primary and secondary soil succession. To achieve this, researchers undertake site-specific studies to identify potential plant species for use in the restoration process. In some cases, heavy soil contamination from coal or metal mining may necessitate expensive site repairs, such as excavation, removal of contaminated soil to secure landfills, and topsoil filling. Alternatively, bioremediation or phytoremediation techniques, which employ plants or other biological methods to extract, degrade, or sequester toxic substances from soil and rubbish heaps, can treat polluted soil.

The ability of a plant species to thrive in a given environment and the characteristics of the substrate will determine how well the mine waste dumps can be restored. To avoid plant mortality during the eco-restoration of the Tirap Colliery's mine OB, researchers screened plant species on-site that could survive the stressful conditions of the mine OB. Indigenous plant species were chosen because they are expected to withstand extreme stress. Thirty-six plant species from 20 different families in the herbaceous, liane, shrub, and tree groups were screened. Axonopus, Saccharum spontaneum, and the commercially significant essential-oil-producing plants Cymbopogon winterianus Jowitt and C. flexuosus were found to be the most robust herbaceous plant species. These plants survived the stressful conditions of mine OB because of the nature of their fibrous root systems. In several mines, researchers found that Gmelina arborea and Dalbergia sissoo tree species and Cassia strata and Sesbania rostrata shrub species were resistant to mine OB stress.

The mine OB disposal site had an acidic pH, no biological activity, and no true soil properties (pH 2.0). Moreover, it had significantly higher trace metal contents than unmined soil. Under these unfavourable conditions, plant species require an extended period to mature, leading to serious ecological damage. Planting herbaceous monocots with fibrous root systems such as citronella, lemongrass, Saccharum spontaneum, lianes, and shrub species can help improve the unfavourable mining OB habitat of Tirap Colliery. The current effort to screen and simultaneously plant multiple plant species will be beneficial in recovering the denuded region of high-sulfide mining OB and achieving long-term sustainable eco-restoration.

5. INTRODUCTION OF PLANT GROWTH-PROMOTING BACTERIA IN MINE DUMPS

Mining waste dumps can be transformed into thriving ecosystems by using bioengineered Plant Growth-Promoting Bacteria (PGPB) that modify the soil to promote plant growth. The soil is a complex ecosystem comprising diverse microorganisms, including bacteria, fungi, actinomycetes, protozoa, and algae. Bacteria make up a significant portion of the soil's total cell population, with only about 1% of these bacteria being culturable. The composition of the soil's microbial community is influenced by factors such as temperature, moisture, salt content, chemical composition, and the presence of plants.

PGPB can be used as a biocontrol agent to enhance plant growth by directly or indirectly affecting plant development. Direct effects may include improved resource acquisition and altered plant hormone levels, while indirect effects involve reducing the inhibitory effects of pathogenic agents on plant growth and development. Bioengineered bacteria can promote plant development by aiding resource acquisition through various mechanisms such as nitrogen fixation, iron sequestration, or phosphate stabilisation.

In mining waste dumps, PGPB can be introduced to modify the soil and promote the growth of various plants. This can significantly impact the restoration of these areas and the creation of thriving ecosystems. By introducing bacteria that improve resource acquisition and reduce the negative effects of pathogens, plants can grow more effectively and ultimately transform the barren landscape into a vibrant ecosystem. This approach holds great promise for sustainable eco-restoration efforts in mining-impacted areas.

6. SCOPE OF BIOENGINEERING ON MINE WATER TREATMENT

In the mining industry, there is a growing interest in using bioengineering processes to improve the treatment of water and soil, as well as to filter gaseous effluents and municipal sewage. The accumulation of water in mining sites, whether in specially designed sumps or the dip side region, is a common occurrence that requires treatment before being released into natural water streams in compliance with regulatory requirements. Innovative treatment processes that use biological systems to remove contaminants from the water, such as heavy metals and organic compounds are being developed to address this issue. One of the approaches used in treating mine water discharge and effluent is the use of Mine Water Discharge Points (MDTP) and Effluent Treatment Plants (ETP). These are specialised facilities developed in mining sites to manage and treat the water and waste products produced in the mine workshop, including grease, oil, and other contaminants. The use of these facilities is an effective way of removing contaminants from the water, with the added benefit of reducing the negative impact of mining activities on the environment.

The bioengineering process has also been applied to soil remediation, which involves the treatment of contaminated soils to remove or neutralise pollutants. In mining sites, soil contamination often occurs due to heavy metals, trace elements, and other harmful chemicals, which can leach into the environment and cause serious environmental damage. Bioremediation techniques that use bacteria and fungi to break down the contaminants have been developed to mitigate this problem. The use of bioengineered microorganisms is particularly effective in removing heavy metals from contaminated soil by using the natural metabolic processes of these microorganisms to immobilise or transform the contaminants into less harmful forms.

Overall, the use of bioengineering processes in the mining industry has the potential to significantly reduce the environmental impact of mining activities while also promoting sustainable practices. By leveraging the natural processes of biological systems, it is possible to treat mining water, soil, and waste products in an effective and environmentally friendly way.

7. CONCLUSION

A modification to a single component within a biological system can have unforeseen effects on the larger ecosystem or specific species due to these systems' intricate, interconnected nature, which allows for cascading impacts. These technologies must be ecologically sound, or alternative mitigation strategies must be implemented to meet the increasing demands for environmental sustainability. As environmental and resource concerns become more pressing, biotechnology will undoubtedly become more widely utilised, and novel technologies will be developed and embraced. For specific applications of metal extraction, bio hydrometallurgy may be considered due to certain technical factors such as favourable mineralogy or the potential to extract value from previously uneconomical materials.

REFERENCES

1) Anna Birjak, Alena Walmsley, Nicole Anderson, Jon Missen and Mohan Yellishetty (2020) Field-scale assessment of artificial topsoil: A Victorian coal mine experience
2) Climate Finance Funding Flows and Opportunities, What Gets Measured Gets Financed, The Rockefeller Foundation; Boston Consulting Group (November 2022)
3) Eds. Roberto C. Villas Boas, Débora Shields, Šlavko Solar, Paul Anciaux, Güven Önal: A Review on Indicators of Sustainability: for the mineral extraction industries XXIII. International Mineral Processing Congress, Istanbul 2006.
4) Gerrit Becker, Luca Bennici, Anamika Bhargava, Andrea Del Miglio, Jeffrey Lewis, and Pankaj Sachdeva; The green IT revolution: A blueprint for CIOs to combat climate change; McKinsey Quarterly (September 2022).
5) J. Dowarah (2009) Eco-restoration of a high-sulphur coal mine overburden dumping site in northeast India: A case study. J. Earth Syst. Sci. 118, No. 5, pp. 597–608
6) How will ESG performance shape your future? Climate Change and Sustainability Services (CCaSS), Fifth global institutional investor survey, July 2020.
7) Lucy Pérez, Vivian Hunt, Hamid Samandari, Robin Nuttall, and Krysta Biniek, Does ESG really matter – and why McKinsey Quarterly (Aug 2022).
8) The Bio Revolution, Innovations transforming economies, societies, and our lives McKinsey Global Institute (May 2020).
9) T. Norgate*, N. Haque. Energy and greenhouse gas impacts of mining and mineral processing operations Journal of Cleaner Production 18 (2010) 266–274
10) Xinhui Li, Shaogang Lei, Feng Liu and Weizhong Wang, Analysis of Plant and Soil Restoration Process and Degree of Refuse Dumps in Open-Pit Coal Mining Areas; International Journal of Environmental Research and Public Health; 17 March 2020
11) Vlado Vivoda and Deanna Kemp, How do national mining industry associations compare on sustainable development? The Extractive Industries and Society, June 2018.